THE BUZZ ON ™

EXERCISE & FITNESS

Rusty Fischer

Paige Waehner

LF LEBHAR-FRIEDMAN BOOKS

NEW YORK · CHICAGO · LOS ANGELES · LONDON · PARIS · TOKYO

The Buzz On Exercise & Fitness

Lebhar-Friedman Books
425 Park Avenue
New York, NY 10022

Published by Lebhar-Friedman Books
Lebhar-Friedman Books is a company of Lebhar-Friedman, Inc.

Printed in the United States of America

Library of Congress Cataloging in Publication Data on file at the Library of Congress

ISBN: 0-86730-856-7

Produced by Progressive Publishing
Editor: John Craddock; Creative Director: Nancy Lycan; Art Director: Angela Connolly
Editorial Contributors: Carolyn Herr, Chandra Beal, Claudine Williams, Daniel Tarker, Deborah Blachor, Dennie Kuhn, Emilie L. Perreault, Jennifer R. Schroeder, Kimberly Ripley, Lisa Carattini, Lindsay Baker, Mark Miller, Megan Costa, Melesa Hamer, Sara Shephard, Stephen Chaleff, Steve Theunissen, Suzanne Giorgi, Tonyia Leet Gray, Paul Love
Designers: Lanette Fitzpatrick, David Womble, Linda Rodriguez, Rena Bracey, Marco Echevarria, Vivian Torres
Production Managers: Mike Bilicki, John Craddock III

Visit our Web site at lfbooks.com

THE BUZZ ON™

EXERCISE & FITNESS

ACKNOWLEDGMENTS

The authors dutifully wish to thank the following for their contributions to this book:

The freelance writers and researchers who helped make this book come together, namely: Carolyn Herr, Chandra Beal, Claudine Williams, Daniel Tarker, Deborah Blachor, Dennie Kuhn, Emilie L. Perreault, Jennifer R. Schroeder, Kimberly Ripley, Lisa Carattini, Lindsay Baker, Mark Miller, Megan Costa, Melesa Hamer, Sara Shephard, Stephen Chaleff, Steve Theunissen, Suzanne Giorgi, Tonyia Leet Gray, and Paul Love.

Haythum Raafat Khalid, who has graciously allowed us to use the quotes found in this book, which also appear on his Web site, Famous Quotations Network: http://www.famous-quotations.com.

Chris White, several of whose Top-5 lists appear in this book and who was a countless inspiration for those that don't! Chris is owner of TopFive.com, at http://www.topfive.com.

THE BUZZ ON
EXERCISE & FITNESS

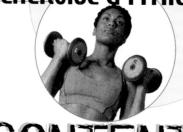

CONTENTS

intro

FITNESS FANATiCS

E xercise? Phooey. And fitness? No, thanks. (Wait a minute, aren't they the same thing?) After all, who the heck needs them? You were a star on the track team back in high school, right kid? Or the captain of the college football team, huh stud? Perhaps you played dynamite hoops or led awesome cheers, Buffy. Or maybe you even fenced or played lacrosse, Senator. However you did it, as an active teen and then an athletic young adult, you burned enough calories each day to down your weight in Gatorade, Power Bars, Big Macs, Snickers, and then some. (Carbo-loading is the proper term, correct?)

But now your twenties are slowly becoming a thing of the past and the only organized sport you play is that weekend game of poker with your buddies. That cushy desk job you played four years worth of college ball on a scholarship to land may mean less stress on your tendons and joints, but when the only exercise you get each day is walking back and forth to the water cooler, is it any wonder that your waist, rear, and thighs are expanding right along with your 401(k) plan?

BETTER BODIES OR BUST!

So *now* who needs exercise and fitness? Well, the fact is, we all do. You don't have to be Richard Simmons to know that regular exercise and the proper diet are two of the biggest keys to unlocking a longer, healthier, happier life. (Plenty of money doesn't hurt, either.) Exercise releases endorphins, makes you sweat, decreases your body weight, and increases your chance of making it to retirement—alive.

True, if this is your first time down the road of sports drinks, exercise equipment, locker rooms, and leotards, the task of starting a regular exercise and fitness program can be quite daunting. What gym should you join, if you join one at all? What are the best shoes for walking? What about rock climbing? How much water should you drink? Is bottled better than tap? Where the heck does that jock strap go?

But don't let the hype intimidate you. The fact is, all you need to get started on the road to a healthier, happier *you* is a strong sense of commitment and a little common sense. Okay, sure, your gym is called Bobby's, not Bally's. Perhaps your leotards came from a thrift shop, not "the body" shop. And maybe you're drinking Kool-Aid instead of Gatorade. Does that make your sweat any less salty than the next guy or your heart beat any less stronger than the next gal?

Heck, no. Look at it this way: In *Rocky 4,* our raw-egg swilling, grammatically incorrect hero had to go up against Drago, a Russian mega-man who had every piece of scientific and technological training equipment known to modern man. If they could manufacture it, he had it: steroids, power shakes,

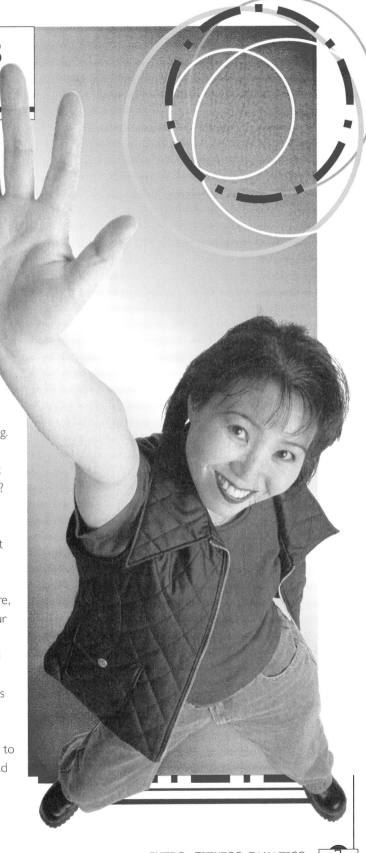

electronic jock straps, the Stairmaster to beat all Stairmasters. What did Rocky have? A musty barn with some rocks, a log, and a really bad fur-lined jacket.

Who won? Our man, Rocky, of course.

Why? Because he had a whole lot of heart and a ton of common sense. (Not to mention, he was the star of the movie.) So if Rocky can beat Superman, the least you can do is climb into those thrift shop leotards and head down to Bobby's Gym with your homemade sports drink.

Go ahead, it'll do your body good.

THE BUZZ ON FITNESS

TOP-5
REASONS TO READ THIS BOOK

5 It costs a lot less than that Nautilus thingamajig you see on TV during your midnight snack each night.

4 Your aerobics instructor said you needed to bring a "step" for next time.

3 *The Buzz On Laziness & Sloth* isn't out yet.

2 The doctor said you needed a little more fiber in your diet.

1 It'll give you something to do at the gym.

TRICEPS TIMELINE, OR: SWEATIN' TO THE (REALLY) OLDIES!

Take a brief tour through the hot and heavy history of exercise and fitness with our convenient Triceps Timeline. From prehistoric stone free weights to the latest ab cruncher offered on those late-night infomercials, it's all here. Just follow the bouncing medicine ball.

HISTORICAL MOMENTS IN EXERCISE & FITNESS

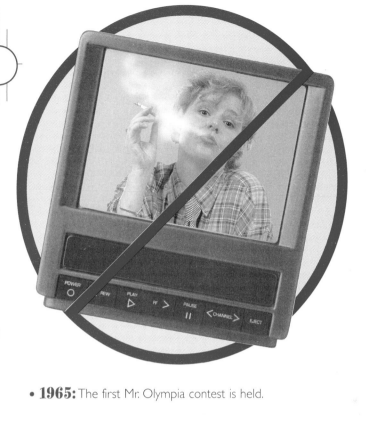

- **1920:** Dr. John Harvey Kellog markets America's first soy food products.

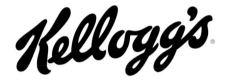

- **1961:** Weight Watchers holds its first meeting in Queens, NY.

- **1962:** Bally's opens its first health club.

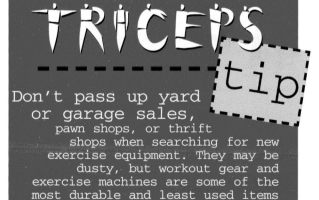

TRICEPS tip

Don't pass up yard or garage sales, pawn shops, or thrift shops when searching for new exercise equipment. They may be dusty, but workout gear and exercise machines are some of the most durable and least used items available second-hand.

- **1965:** The first Mr. Olympia contest is held.

- **1966:** Gold's Gym opens its first gym.

- **1970:** Arnold Schwarzenegger wins his first Mr. Olympia title.

- **1970:** Cigarette ads are banned from television and radio.

- **1972:** Nike creates their "swoosh" logo.

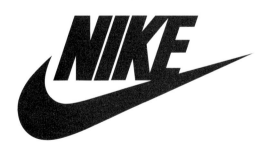

- **1977:** Jazzercise becomes a popular form of exercise.

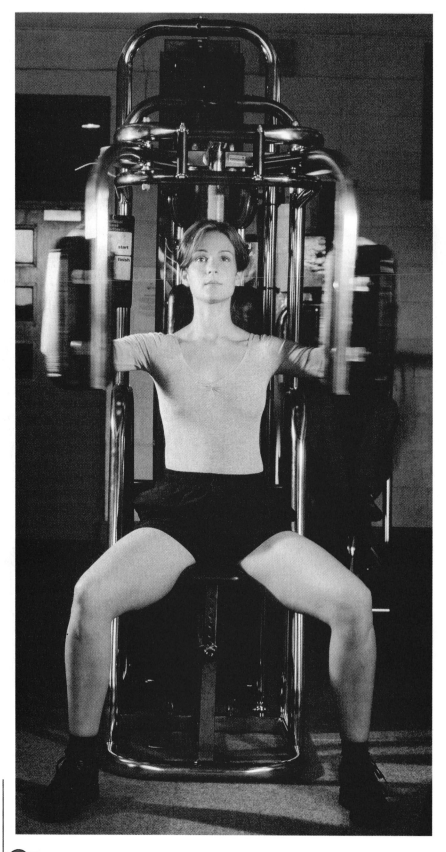

- **1978:** The Soloflex Muscle Machine was first introduced.

- **1980s:** During the '80s, going to health clubs becomes a trend.

- **1982:** Jane Fonda releases her first in a series of workout videos.

- **1982:** Liposuction was introduced to American cosmetic surgeons.

- **1983:** Aerobics and Fitness Association is founded.

- **1985:** President's Council on Physical Fitness opens.

- **1985:** Nike releases the first line of "Air Jordan" shoes.

- **1988:** Richard Simmons comes out with *Sweatin' to the Oldies.*

- **1990s:** Spandex becomes a popular type of exercise clothing.

- **1991:** Lee Haney wins his record 8th consecutive Mr. Olympia title.

- **1986:** Suzanne Somers does the ThighMaster infomercials.

- **1986:** The first line of Bowflex machines is developed.

• **1987:** After doing a video with Prince, Sheena Easton popularizes washboard abs for women.

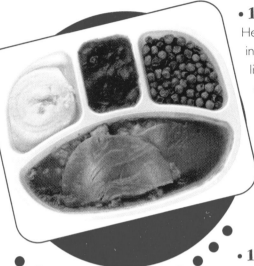

• **1988:** Healthy Choice introduces its line of frozen dinners.

• **1994:** Richard Simmons introduces Deal-A-Meal.

• **1995:** ESPN launches the *Body By Jake* television workout show.

• **1997:** NordicTrack unveils the Ellipse exercise machine.

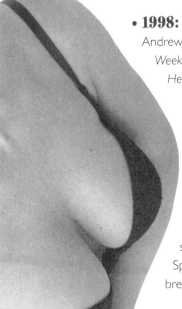

• **1998:** Health guru Andrew Weil publishes *8 Weeks to Optimum Health.*

• **1998:** Tae-Bo becomes popularized.

• **1999:** Rumors swarm that teen pop sensation Britney Spears had her breasts enlarged.

• **2000:** Adventure racing becomes popular.

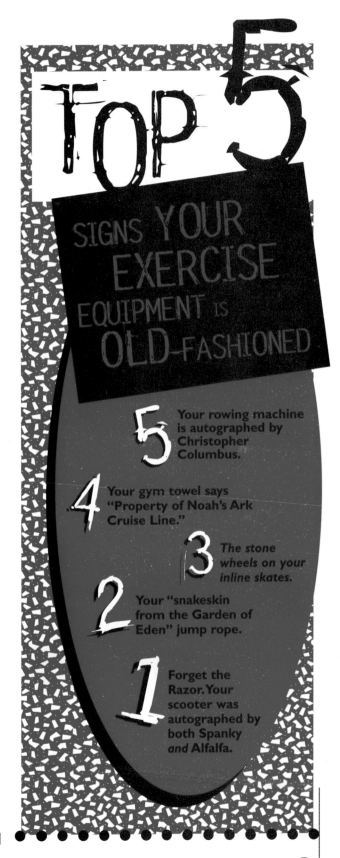

TOP 5

SIGNS YOUR EXERCISE EQUIPMENT IS OLD-FASHIONED

5 Your rowing machine is autographed by Christopher Columbus.

4 Your gym towel says "Property of Noah's Ark Cruise Line."

3 The stone wheels on your inline skates.

2 Your "snakeskin from the Garden of Eden" jump rope.

1 Forget the Razor. Your scooter was autographed by both Spanky *and* Alfalfa.

1 ASS—ESSMENT

Before you begin any regular program filled with exercise and fitness, not to mention blood, sweat, tears, and whining, it is best to get a proper ass-essment of your current situation. Are you a former steroid junkie who's fallen off the wagon? A current beauty queen who's been hitting the all-you-can-eat buffets a little too hard lately? Or just a regular Joe or Jane trying to make it up the stairs each night without having to stop halfway up and wheeze for a few minutes?

Either way, there are a few hard facts to face first. One: Unless you're already Tom Cruise, you probably won't end up looking like him after a few weeks at the gym. (Especially if your name is Tom Booze.) Two: No matter what those hotties on the cover of that 3-Minute Abs video might say, it will probably take you a lot longer to get six-pack abs of your own. (Especially if you're downing a real six-pack after your workout each night!)

And, finally, no matter how hard it might be, you'll have to take a long, hard look in the mirror and decide exactly what areas need improving. (And which others can only be helped by surgery.)

MEASURING UP,
OR: THE LONGEST YARD (STICK)

Did you know that your scale is a highly unreliable method of measuring your fitness? Think of your scale, wherever it is right now, as a squat, mindless little dictator telling you on its terms what a lump you are. Now think of your scale mashed under the back tire of your car. The little needle has snapped in two—miniature gleaming springs dangle from the cracked carcass. Feels good, doesn't it? Go ahead. Free at last.

The reason a scale is so unreliable as a sole source of fitness info is that it can determine only one statistic: your weight, in pounds or kilograms. It delivers this one statistic, indifferent to height, body shape, muscle-to-fat ratio, or any other factors important to a healthy weight. The number you see in the scale window is only conveying part of the story; on the other hand, if you can't read the scale over your belly, that does tell you something. And for most people it's true that you set your goals for losing X pounds in the next three days before the wedding or reunion or whatever.

Still, there are far more trustworthy ways of measuring the health of your body and its functions.

MEASURE YOUR BODY FAT

Healthy body fat for women should be between 18 and 25 percent. To keep their bodies healthy, men require 10 to 18 percent. Body fat refers to what percentage of your total weight is actually fat, and not bones, skin, organs, water, and other important parts

you shouldn't shed or sell. Any doctor or clinic can perform a skin fold body composition test, in which a fold of your skin is measured for thickness. An instrument known as a caliper measures the fat under your skin at your abdomen, back of the arm, thigh, hip, or the back of your shoulder. Not after a workout though.

> *"He who does not mind his belly will hardly mind anything else."*
> —Samuel Johnson

Fluid transfer during workouts affects caliper readings. This is better than that dumb scale. Now you know what your percentage of body fat is. Is it between 18 and 25 percent? If your number is too high, you now know by how much, and can begin to think of your healthy number as a goal.

Want to know something kind of unsettling? Keeping in mind that the female body needs a minimum of 18 percent body fat to function at peak, except in some professional athletes, consider the body fat percentages of Jennifer Aniston, 8.49 percent; Mariah Carey, 5.39; Cindy Crawford, 9.37. Teri Hatcher's body fat percentage is a terrifying 4.78! It's comforting to know that, even if your number is high, you may be healthier than these famous women.

TIPS ON MEASURING BODY PARTS

1. **Don't use a yardstick.**
2. **Use millimeters, it sounds smaller.**
3. **Suck it in before measuring.**
4. **Round to the lowest inch/foot.**
5. **Lie flat while measuring flabby areas.**

MEASURE YOUR FITNESS

You can find hundreds of people all around the world with high body fat, who are at the same time, technically, physically fit. Somewhat overweight people who are otherwise fit are less vulnerable to illness and disease than thin people who don't exercise. Well, imagine that. Don't get too excited, though, until you can pass all of the tests for physical fitness:

Endurance tests measure your aerobic fitness. They test how fast your heart beats at rest and during strenuous exercise. This indicates how many extra times your heart needs to beat in order to deliver enough oxygen to support your activity—like walking to your car or getting out of bed.

If you find yourself gasping like a fish after tackling a flight of stairs, or if you can't survive the rigors of a 12-minute run, you're most likely not aerobically fit. Your poor heart can't keep up with your needs for oxygen. Also important is how quickly your heart returns to normal rhythm; the more time it takes for you to recover, the deeper in oxygen debt your heart is.

Strength and power tests measure your strength against resistance, your top speed, and the power of your sprints and jumps. Your ability to lift weight, pump your legs against the ground, or defy gravity is an excellent means of measuring strength. Sumo wrestlers and champion weight lifters rely on their strength above all else; these athletes are among the largest, and heaviest, in the world. It is not unusual at all for a pro lifter to weigh 300 pounds; this number alone is meaningless.

Flexibility tests measure the capacity of a joint to move through its full range of motion. If you stretch every day, or if you practice yoga, flexibility is a daily part of your life. Reaching for the remote control should not make you grunt! Neither should touching your own toes, scratching your back, or moving the seat back in any car. Flexibility allows your body to move more efficiently, promotes toning and good posture, and reduces muscle cramping, injury, and stiffness.

MEASURE YOUR PORTIONS

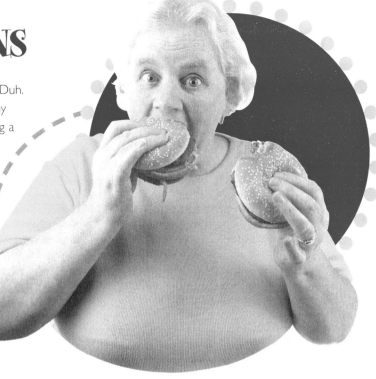

If you eat too much, you will gain weight. Duh. Healthy portions will help your body; unhealthy portions will weigh you down. Start by keeping a journal, writing down everything you eat, without making any changes. These records help you see, in black and white, what you are feeding your face, and how much. Usually, you will be able to isolate problem times (after 7 p.m. snacking), deficiencies (yeah, right, you ate six servings of veggies today), or weaknesses (birthday cake at the office three times a week), and then you'll be able to conquer the almighty bad habit! It's chilling to think that you might have bad eating habits without realizing it, or even enjoying it.

Once you have isolated these evils, and conquered them, you can begin to enter the mine-laden territory of everyday eating. A weighty aspect of everyday eating is portion size. Restaurant portions of pasta are twice as big as ten years ago, for a comparable price. If you were to go back in time to 1980, you would find a large order of fast food fries to be roughly the size of today's medium. Now, if you don't "Humongous size" your meal, the minimum wage server thinks you're cheap!

The country is eating more, there's a big emphasis on value (want to "biggie up" for fifty cents?), and it is hardly surprising that the rest of the nation has influenced your eating habits. Need proof? Consider the following:

• Eating an entire box of macaroni and cheese is not a portion. A single portion is however much fills the inside of a standard coffee mug.

• A single serving of peanut butter on a slice of bread is about the size of a golf ball.

• A portion of chicken or steak, three ounces, is about the size of a deck of cards.

Consider what's on the end of your fork very carefully before you stick it in your craw; it's a little too late once you've swallowed it. Find an easy way to measure the food on your plate, one that you can use daily and is as simple as checking your watch.

If you concentrate on measuring up to your own standards, and your own goals of becoming healthy, the scale will never haunt you again. As a final reminder to how useless the scale truly is, think of a 160-pound woman who has begun to work out and is enjoying the feel of her clothes more every day. She's feeling motivated and inspired, not to mention confident. After a month of feeling this way, she makes the mistake of stepping on a damnable scale. In no uncertain terms, it tells her that she has not lost any weight!

Perhaps she doesn't know that muscle weighs 22 percent more than fat, and takes up less space, and that she has been steadily replacing fat on her body with muscle. She has never felt better in her life, but the scale is stupid.

Look: She's backing her car out of the driveway now. Take *that*, you stupid scale!

MIRROR MADNESS, OR: FACING (FAT) FACTS

"Mirror, mirror, on the wall . . ." Imagine what it must be like to dread the sight of a mirror, to fear and despise it, for no other reason than it remembers the condition of your body. It's not the mirror's fault; you simply fear and despise your own body and the very sight of it.

When inspecting yourself in the mirror, your unwilling eye is immediately drawn to your belly, thighs, and ass. The good mood you were in begins to fade. You curse the mirror silently, because a notion you have embraced for years is cast off momentarily by the hateful reflective surface! The notion is this: If I ignore it, it will go away, and it will all be okay.

A mirror can only show the truth, so here is a new notion: The longer you ignore it, the bigger and more dangerous it will get. The truth hurts.

Does it have to?

FEAR AND LOATHING (IN THE MIRROR)

It is how the truth impacts you that is really important as you stand gazing into the mirror. The fact is, you think you're fat and ugly. Is this what the mirror is telling you, or is it what your husband's been telling you for years? Is it how you feel when you look at Cindy Crawford? Or, most likely of all, is it all you?

You have options.

One option is to hate your body, and the burden it has become in life! You can live by forever selecting clothes a few sizes too big, ordering tacos for three, and staying on the dark side of mirrors. Exercise is difficult and demanding; your body is way too out of shape for that!

Besides, you hardly ever need energy anyway. Making jokes at your own expense, about your blubber butt or twin chins, may even disguise some of the disgust you feel when trying to find a picture in the entire photo album that you actually don't loathe! You are convinced that others perceive you in the same way you perceive yourself, but you make this assumption based on your reflection, which is tainted by your

TRICEPS tip

Be realistic. Don't focus on exercises you find unpleasant or uncomfortable. Choosing activities you enjoy will help you stick with your program. Plan for success.

opinion of yourself! Now you not only dread the mirror, you also have developed an irrational paranoia of other humans as well!

Obviously, since ignoring the truth has worked so well in the past, it seems you are determined to continue on this course, and to endure any pains you inflict on yourself in the process. These are your choices, and this is your body.

DEPRIVATION
NATION

Another way to punish your hateful body is to stop feeding it. Even though the mirror always tells the truth, you can convince yourself that it lies. This body had better get thin, and now! Since food is converted into fat, cutting out the food will cut out the fat, a reasonable hypothesis! Except—food is also converted into other things of slight importance, like blood, bone, hair, energy, muscle tissue, and defense against disease. Like any other machine, the body will stall if it is denied fuel, coolant, lubrication, or pretty much any other fluid in the owner's manual. The moment you fail to fuel your body, it stops burning calories to conserve vital energy; you have placed your body in "starvation mode," a handy condition for hunter-gatherers, but a tad counterproductive for weight loss!

The mirror is still reflecting a fatty! How can this be, when you've even stopped having your period?

Lately you hate the mirror even more, but since you are so close to the perfect size, you think you can probably endure.

Why are you enduring? Why aren't you living?

THE TRUTH HURTS?

The mirror speaks the truth, but you are lying to yourself. You are far from ugly. Look at your body; don't look away! See how your chest rises and falls without any thought. Raise your arms, flex them, concentrate on the feeling in your muscles; they glow even after this small attention. Place your feet shoulder-width apart, and, keeping your back straight, bend your knees to a 90-degree angle. Notice anything? Those are your quadricep muscles, long-neglected, eager to be called to duty! Breathe deeply, taste the air, listen to your heartbeat. Think what you could do with your muscles awake and ready! Imagine the invincibility a strong heart could lend you! Your body is not ugly, it is awe-inspiring and unique, and if you love it, you will learn to care for it. If you learn to care for it, there is nothing your body will not do for you.

FUEL FOR THOUGHT

Caring for your body means finding out, just as you would with a new car or lawn mower, what the best fuel might be for a machine such as yours, and how much is best for optimal performance. If you don't know, ask someone who does! They will tell you to drink a liter of water a day and eat six to eight servings of veggies and four to six servings of fruit, for a start. No, the lettuce on a Big Mac does not count as a veggie.

Caring for your body also means exercising it. Even a dog gets a daily walk if the owner is attentive in the least! Try to remember your life before you discovered the automobile. You rode your bike or skateboarded everywhere; you conquered the playground on a daily basis and rarely found yourself out of breath or energy. Your body needs about 30 minutes per day of huffing and puffing. And not from smoking, either.

This will not be easy. You must change your life and the way you eat forever. You must pass up fat eight times out of ten. And you must exercise your body. This, ultimately, is the truth you are facing in the mirror; this truth is the most difficult to face. Change, or face the mirror every day as a lifelong adversary.

The mirror may be reflecting your body, but what are your emotions telling you? Are you loving your chubby hips, or hating your thin ones? Most compelling of all, is there a way to look into the mirror and respect what you see because it's yours, instead of comparing it with the reflections of others?

Don't you see? Simply by eating properly and exercising a moderate amount every day, you are doing something positive, and this will change the way you see yourself in the mirror. Getting a new hairdo or buying a new wardrobe draws you to the mirror because you want to see the positive results of your effort!

The more effort you put in, the more positive the results, the less effort you put in, the guiltier and more negative your perspective. Worst of all, the less you do for yourself, the more you berate your body, the more you punish yourself over your appearance—the more you will hate your reflection! This is a vicious cycle so perfect, it's nearly a cliché! It's not about your fat ass after all; it's about your fragile, paper-thin self-image.

There are people all over the world with less-than-perfect, less-than-healthy bodies who adore what they see when they encounter a mirror. The reflections of others are meaningless to these wise, confident heroes; they know that since their own choices have shaped their bodies, and they respect these choices, they do not shy away from the mirror. They not only accept the mirror's truth, they embrace it, because they are proud of life's accomplishments, and proud of themselves.

Perhaps you can find a middle ground between changing the way you live, thus changing your body, and changing the way you accept the truth the mirror has to tell.

Mirror, mirror, on the wall . . .

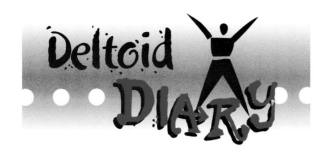

Reflection Deception

Let's face it—mirrors lie. They plot and connive with one another until they have us completely convinced we look like hell. Adrianna, a young model-wannabe sales clerk, discovered this conspiracy while retailing in a haute couture boutique. One

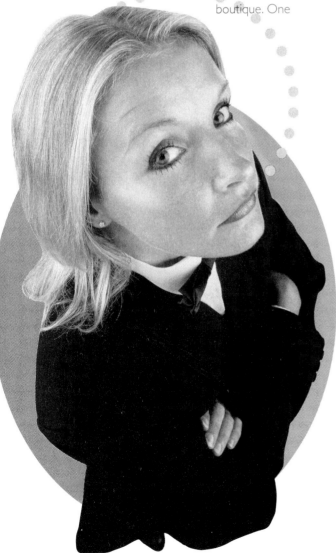

evening, while straightening the dressing rooms, she was privy to a conversation whose origin took serious sleuthing to discover.

"Distort them in the ass," she heard.

"Hello?"

Nobody answered.

"Mess with the lighting. That makes them look dimpled and pale."

"Hello?" she said louder. "Who's in here?"

Again, no reply.

"I love to watch the skinny ones," another voice chimed in. "They strut and pose and turn to every imaginable angle to catch all views of

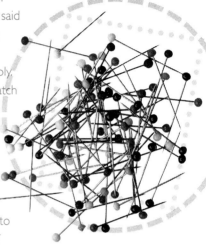

themselves. Then they go out to the showroom and the first thing they ask is 'Does it make me look fat?' I can't stand those types. Play with the lighting. Distort those wispy wenches and make them look like they've put on a few pounds."

"I can't. I'm cracked. One of those larger ladies banged into me with her handbag when she bent over to get the hanger. There really wasn't enough room in here for her. It was an accident."

Was it? No, it couldn't be. Holy cow, it was! Those mirrors were talking. They were conversing back and forth amongst themselves and deciding how to put instant fear into the minds of unsuspecting women.

Adrianna feared she was losing her mind.

"Breathe deeply, you're not losing your mind," she began whispering softly to herself.

Tiptoeing to the first changing stall, Adrianna parked herself on the carpet—nearly screamed from sitting on a straight pin, but was able to refrain herself—then settled in to continue eavesdropping on these "reflections."

"Pssst, down here—it's me, in changing room #3. Had a real beauty in here today. Phew! She stunk of

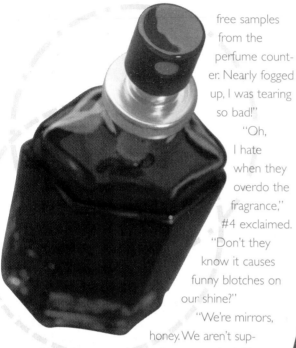

free samples from the perfume counter. Nearly fogged up, I was tearing so bad!"

"Oh, I hate when they overdo the fragrance," #4 exclaimed. "Don't they know it causes funny blotches on our shine?"

"We're mirrors, honey. We aren't supposed to be concerned with the way we look. They only look at us because they're concerned about the way they look—they're so vain!"

"And to think—we get to see them in the flesh, and they don't even know it!"

"I don't think they care. Hello? We're mirrors—get it? We're nothing more than reflective glass."

"But we can make them feel good or we can make them feel bad."

"How do we decide which one to do?" asked #7, a new installation.

"Well, that all depends," #9 replied. "I like to first hear how she treats the sales help. If she's sweet and gracious and treats her with respect, then I tend to alter my lighting just enough to buffer her most prominent flaws. I mean, if she's a nice person, why make her feel bad for something Mother Nature did? And if she's a snob, and is rude to the clerk, then it's time to pull out all the stops."

"What do you mean?" #7 asked in her most naive voice.

"I mean, if she can't be kind and considerate, then neither can we. If she's a skinny little thing, and a bit neurotic about it at that, then I can adjust myself to make it look like she's gained weight. I can make the

shopper appear to have blotchy skin, a saggy butt, stretch marks far more pronounced than they really are—you name it!"

"But that isn't very nice—even if she was rude. Maybe she's just having a bad day," #7 added.

"Look, sweetheart, if you want to fit in here, I suggest you develop our work ethics. Rude is rude, and we don't allow anyone we work with to be treated that way."

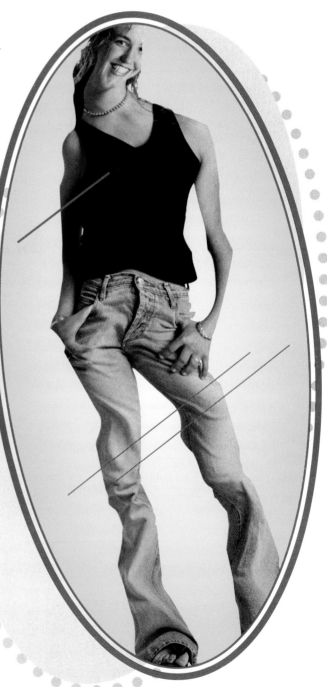

"But the clerks don't know we talk—do they?"

"Of course not. That would make all hell break loose. Rather than using us as reflective glass, they would invite droves of people to parade by us and gawk. Then they'd gawk at themselves, and we'd have to endure all kinds of abuse. People would adjust their private parts, comb their hair—they'd perform all sorts of indignities. It would be disgusting."

"Oh, the absolutely most disgusting thing I ever watched was a grown woman squeezing a zit. It flew all over me, and no one came to clean me up until nearly eleven o'clock that night!" the haughty #2 chimed in.

Adrianna still felt weak from the understanding that she was listening to a conversation between a bunch of mirrors. Uncertain what they might do if she proclaimed her presence, she remained sitting quietly, plotting how and when to take her leave.

"Should I decide to inform my coworkers of my eavesdropping, they would undoubtedly tell me to leave, so I think I'd better keep my mouth shut," Adrianna thought. "I guess it would sound a bit irrational, wouldn't it?"

Before she could conjure another thought in her disbelieving little mind, she heard what sounded like a roll call in progress.

"Lighting—#1? Are you positive or negative?"

"Positive, sir."

"And what about you, #2?"

"I'm negative, sir. I'm out for thighs, sir."

"Good, that's good, #2. Do them in with dimples, sags—throw in a little scaly skin, too."

"Scaly skin, sir. That's good."

And so this continued until each and every mirror in the entire dressing room had provided the head mirror with a description of what they would project for images the next day. Adrianna was appalled. She was completely aghast! This was worse than security cameras or peep holes in the dressing rooms!

"But wait—this is crazy. These aren't people I'm referring to—these are mirrors. This mirror madness is really driving me insane," Adrianna whispered out loud to herself.

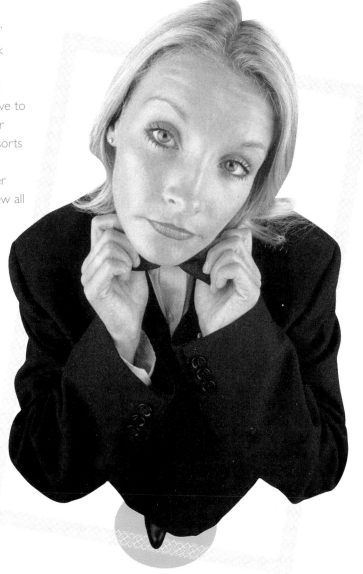

She slowly rose to her feet, and staggered back out onto the shop floor. She busied herself by straightening a few racks and hanging up a few returns. After a little while she was approached by a portly older woman.

"May I try these on, dear?"

"Four items?" she politely asked. "Yes, come right this way."

As the lady closed the door to her private little cubicle, Adrianna pictured the image of chubby thighs and upper arm flab. She then imagined the fun those mirrors were having with this specimen.

And she wished she'd been a fly on the wall—or maybe the mirror—to witness the critique!

PROPORTION DISTORTION RANT, OR: "I LOVE MYSELF, I HATE MYSELF!"

What would you do, what would you give to be thin? Would you do anything to be a tall, willowy bone rack? So would the average woman. Unfortunately for you, the average American woman is 5'4", weighs 140 pounds, and wears size 14 dresses; one third of all American women wear a size 16 or larger. If you are an average American woman, you will never be a tall, willowy bone rack, even if you are willing to give your very life.

Besides, how did you come to think that her body is better or more attractive than your body? Of course, this is not a notion that you were born with; nor is it likely that your parents would knowingly inflict it upon you (Hollywood moms and dads excepted).

Since you were a little child, something insidious and omnipresent has been persuading you that an average, 5'4" frame with its small-to-medium breasts and fleshy posterior is unnatural, unhealthy, and ungainly. This something has been gaining power, over the last twenty years especially, to warp our most innate principles of beauty and shape.

It's called the media, and it is powerful.

For a while now, we've known that thin people are simply better than average-weight people. It has taken about two decades for the media to cultivate the notion that tremendously thin people are tremendously better than average ones, especially when it comes to women. After all, with 75 percent of American women unhappy with their weight, the diet industry, and its foods, programs, and drugs, among countless other promotions, rakes in over $40 billion each year, and is still growing.

How many diet plans can you name out loud? How many of them have you inflicted on yourself? Jenny Craig, Weight Watchers, Slim-Fast, Metabolife, Fatban, high protein, liquid, grapefruit, cabbage, pasta, grass, feathers! If it's not a food plan, it's a drug; Xenical is selling despite the words of warning about gas with oily

"Ever notice that you never see a man walking down the street with a woman who has a little pot belly and a bald spot."
—Elayne Boosler

discharge. A fenfluramine and phentermine combination was a hot seller for ten years before the Mayo Clinic discovered that fen-phen causes heart valve damage and primary pulmonary hypertension, a potentially fatal progressive disease with no known cure, and often no symptoms! Dieters hope and trust that extreme plans can induce extreme change, and they will pay extreme amounts of money to change themselves.

Quick weight-loss schemes are among the most common consumer frauds, and diet programs have the highest customer dissatisfaction of any service industry. Between 90 percent and 99 percent of reducing diets fail to produce permanent weight loss, and two-thirds of dieters regain the weight within one year. Virtually all regain it within five years, but by then they've saved up enough money to give it another go.

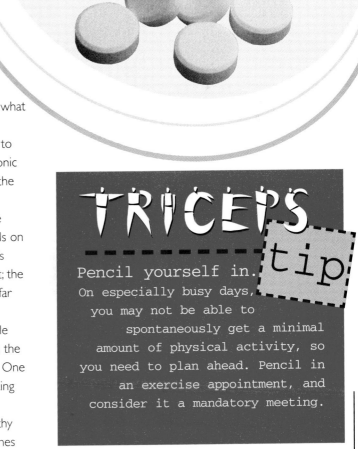

You've met the average woman; you see that you are not alone in your fears or in your struggles. Now meet the ideal woman, who is a model, Miss America, or a screen idol. She is 5'7", weighs 100 pounds, and wears a size 6. You can see her on any magazine cover, movie screen, rock video, or on the fashion runway. If you met her face-to-face, her thinness would alarm you.

Twenty years ago, this ideal weighed only 8 percent less than the average woman, and today she weighs 23 percent less. Don't worry, that's just the media working! Marilyn Monroe wore a size 12, but now, a size 8 is really what you should be reducing for.

Next, the ideal woman should be airbrushed to perfection; cellulite does not sell cosmetics. Electronic alteration can make an ideal woman out of even the most average fare. You thought *Jurassic Park* was impressive? That is not Julia Roberts's body on the cover of the *Pretty Woman* video, and most models on the cover of *Cosmopolitan* appear to be freaks. It is impossible for a human being to be media-perfect; the very models and stars extolled by the media are far from perfect.

Would you risk death to reach an unreachable ideal? Women are dying to be ideal; anorexia has the highest mortality rate of any psychiatric diagnosis. One out of every four college-aged women has an eating disorder because they don't know the difference between a healthy body and an ideal one. A healthy body is challenged every day to empower the genes

TRICEPS tip

Pencil yourself in. On especially busy days, you may not be able to spontaneously get a minimal amount of physical activity, so you need to plan ahead. Pencil in an exercise appointment, and consider it a mandatory meeting.

that it was born with, to be lean and strong, vital and enduring.

An ideal body is a fantasy that makes you feel ashamed of the genes you were born with in a very subliminal and deliberate way.

A psychological study in 1995 found that three minutes spent looking at models in a fashion magazine caused 70 percent of women to feel depressed, guilty, and shameful. Three minutes! How many minutes have

TRICEPS tip

Break it up. Exercise doesn't have to be all at one time or in one session. Busy people can get much the same benefits when they exercise in bits and pieces throughout the day as when they work out in one block of time.

you wasted and suffered through looking at these same models? You may not want to hear this, but you will never be the media's idea of the ideal woman or man, so you may as well concentrate on matters of a little more importance, matters that make you feel the opposite of depressed, guilty, or shameful. Start by looking at the fashions, not the models. The models are only spectacularly paid clothes racks anyway. Imagine how you might feel wearing that exact outfit to an awards banquet in your honor. Picture your sparkling entrance as the applause and cheers of loved ones and coworkers greet you! Hold onto that positive image while you flip through the rest of the magazine. "Try on" as many outfits as you want.

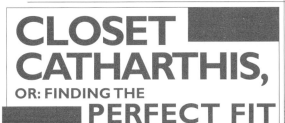

CLOSET CATHARTHIS,
OR: FINDING THE
PERFECT FIT

There is an old rule of thumb that has been used in reference to the cleaning out of closets for eons: "If you haven't worn it in two years—out it goes." Now, for yo-yo dieters and sporadic exercise buffs, this could present a bit of a problem. There are, in fact, many people who hang on to several different sizes of clothing to accommodate the ever changing weight and size of their physiques. However, this isn't always a practical recommendation, as most people's homes have storage restrictions. There just isn't enough room to store years' and years' worth of clothing. And you might as well face it, many things are simply no longer in style. So donate these unwanted articles of clothing. Give them to a friend. Or throw the darned things away—but whatever option you choose, get rid of them!

Closets can reveal a lot about a person's personality. It is also possible to determine a great deal about someone by observing the way she purges her closets and dressers. The tightwad's closet is often filled with nicely tailored clothing. In fact, tightwads often buy extremely high quality clothing. Then they proceed to wear these items for twenty-three years. A woman's closet containing several plaid Pendleton suits is obviously a closet belonging to a tightwad.

The thrift shop junky has a closet that combines a taste for eclectic (in other words tacky) clothing, combined with a need for purchasing inexpensive items. Too creative to simply run to the nearest Wal-Mart for a few new things, this type of person actually enjoys rummaging through these dirty old garments, often scented with cedar and moth balls. An old hippie at heart, this personality type becomes positively ecstatic when discovering a tie-dyed T-shirt and a leather vest sporting a 10-inch long fringe.

It is always fun to compare a man's closet to a woman's closet. This is one of very few areas where a man is generally neater than a woman! Yes, it's the truth. Most men's closets are arranged according to each particular type of clothing. For example, all of their pants hang together, all of their jackets hang together, and all of their shirts hang together. Their shoes (all three functional pairs) are lined neatly on the floor of the closet.

A woman's closet, however, is disguised as a disaster in progress. Nothing hangs uniformly. Belts are slung randomly over the rod, purses are piled on top of one another, and stray blouses and scarves decorate the unmatched heap of shoes on the closet floor. It's almost as if a strong gust of wind blew inside the house, missing all of its contents, and aimed directly for this closet. It's a huge mess.

Dieters and sporadic exercisers usually find that their needs in clothing change as their habits increase or decrease. In the fall and winter, one may be up to two clothing sizes larger than in the spring and summer. It obviously is not cost conscious to expect

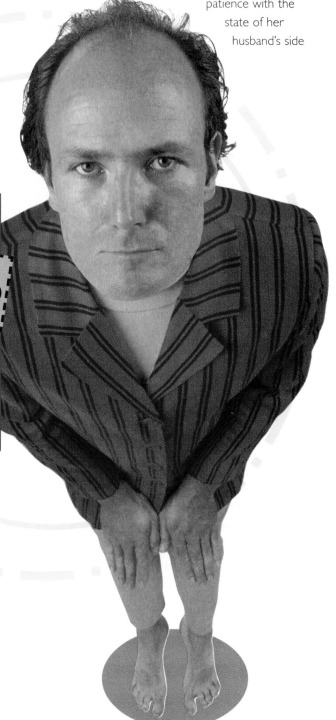

TRICEPS tip

Commit yourself.
You owe it to yourself and your family to be as healthy as you can be. Committing to daily physical activity must be part of your life. Strive—don't just survive!

these folks to get rid of any of these sets of clothing. They would wind up purchasing new ones as their weight fluctuated. They need to invest in alternative methods of storage—or build bigger closets.

A catharsis of a closet is revered almost as highly as the purging of the soul. Items once deemed valuable have lost their glitz and their glitter. They now sit idly, untouched and unused, and await a second life at the hands of another fashion expert. It is refreshing to eliminate items from a closet. It provides a clearer look at what matters most in your world of fashion. It solves the problem of needing some extra space, and you actually wind up with a wonderful excuse to do a little shopping. It doesn't get much better than that!

One hard and fast rule must apply to a closet catharsis. No one, and that is "NO One" with a capital "NO"—should ever purge another person's closet. This happened to a woman in Queens once whose patience with the state of her husband's side of the closet was at an all-time low. Not an untidy man, he simply had an odd taste in fashion. He had a collection of several shimmering, silky shirts that looked as though they were straight out of *Saturday Night Fever*.

His wife could just imagine him strutting his stuff under the disco ball like a much younger John Travolta once strutted. He'd never worn any of the shirts since their marriage (and for this she was eternally grateful!), so she assumed they were of little importance to him. She donated them to their church's thrift shop, where they were sold at $3 each. When her husband discovered them among the missing, he grew frantic. When she finally admitted that she'd been in a cleaning mode and eliminated several things from their closets, he nearly lost his mind.

It seems the shirts didn't just look like they were from *Saturday Night Fever*—they were in fact worn in the hit movie by Travolta himself! Her husband had posted them at online auctions all over the Internet, and was expecting to earn a handsome profit when they sold!

> *"In any closet, you can find it, if it is too small, or out of style, or there is just one of it where there should be two. I am not sure what this is, but an 'F' would only dignify it."*
> —*Anonymous English Professor*

There are a couple of things here that are imperative to remember. First of all, if you fluctuate between heavy and thin, be very frugal when getting rid of clothes. If you have remained the same size for a few years and have no plans of losing (or gaining) additional weight, donate or give away old and unusable clothing.

Thrift shops, church organizations, the Salvation Army, and even some elementary schools are usually more than happy to receive contributions of gently worn clothing.

The most important rule would be this: In addition to strictly adhering to your own side of the closet, do not ever assume your significant other is a gigantic fashion faux pas. What is the reason behind such a statement? It's simple. And it's quite likely you've heard this old adage before. "If you keep it kicking around long enough, it's bound to come back into style."

ALLY McBACKLASH

The trend is real, even if the Hollywood sound bites are not. Of course Ally McBeal isn't going to admit that she's anorexic. After all, she's a lawyer, isn't she?

It was destined to happen, of course. Ever since *Seinfeld* went off the air and we all grew used to seeing somebody or another's butt on *NYPD Blue*, what else was there to talk about at the water cooler on Monday morning?

"Did you see *Friends* last night? What is with Monica? She turned sideways and I thought for a minute she was a lamp. And Rachel? Come on. Does she think she has to keep up with Ally by turning into a ghost herself?"

It's not fair, of course. What celebrities eat, or more importantly *don't* eat, in their personal lives is entirely up to them. In fact, it is *our* fault for holding them up as role models and believing that if *they* look that way, so should we.

Calista Flockhart (Ally McBeal), therefore, has every right to get pissed when Connie Chung asks her if there's a problem or, more pointedly, tells her that she looks "sick." More power to her. Of course, the fact that Chung was right gets lost in the moment.

Which, we must assume, Calista Flockhart's publicists, agents, managers, and close, personal, similarly anorexic friends, who thought up the ploy, most certainly intended.

What gets overlooked, of course, is the fact that we actually *care* that all of those starving starlets look unhealthy. It's not that we begrudge them their obvious talent, beauty, and untold riches. (Okay, of course we do.) Regardless, we won't let that stand in the way of our concern for their safety.

This concern, of course, is a double-edged sword, at least to celebrities. We don't want you to get too thin. That's disgusting. However, just don't get too fat, either. That's even worse.

Remember Alicia Silverstone? That poor thing. Doesn't every teenager grow up, lose her baby fat, grow up a little more, and regain it all as a young adult? Is it her fault she did it in the public eye?

How about Elizabeth Taylor?

The answer is simple, of course. We should all just mind our own business. But how are we supposed to, when the media takes advantage of every slow news day to point out some starlet or another's pointy pelvis, crinkly backbone, or withered face?

After all, in the absence of wars or school shootings, Hollywood has always been a reporter's safest bet.

Yet, why are people so disconcerted at the sight of Calista Flockhart and her teeny-tiny waist, bony knuckles, and hollow cheeks? Thin is in, the problem being that *radically* thin is *radically* in. How much healthier is Ally McBeal than Roseanne Connor was

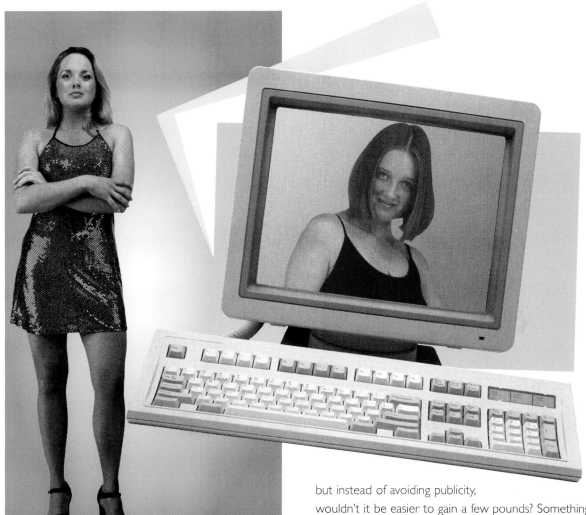

at her scale-splintering heaviest, and how much healthier are her eating habits? Of course, nobody cares about *that* part! Being a healthy woman is hardly a prerequisite for prime time television.

The reason we're worried: Our daughters, sisters, mothers, and lovers don't seem to know the difference between television and real life. Their role models often appear to resemble prisoners of war. They are slowly and relentlessly becoming convinced that emaciated equals elegance.

Calista Flockhart actually pulled out of a *Today* interview because the studio would not promise to avoid the subject of her weight, or lack thereof! She insists she's weary of being plagued with this question, but instead of avoiding publicity, wouldn't it be easier to gain a few pounds? Something that would work: Eating! It isn't only that we can see the bones of Ally, Rachel, Monica, and Daphne through their skin at the elbows; it's the image of starving kids in Africa that seems to leap forth unbidden. Though they are hardly desperate kids, these TV women don't seem to have the energy to improve and strengthen their bodies: The scrawny arms and legs, the large, bony cranium balanced on the fragile stalk of a neck, the little-boy bust—whoever told these women that this is sexy, desirable, or necessary?

Far more popular, worshipped on endless print and Web pages it seems, are bodies like those of the astoundingly fit Carmen Electra, the beautiful and shapely Jennifer Lopez, and the seductive, voluptuous Catherine Zeta-Jones. In comparison to these lean and vital women, the diminutive Calista Flockhart is reminiscent of a shrill and hungry Chihuahua.

2 SCORING GOALS
(WITH GREAT PLANNING)

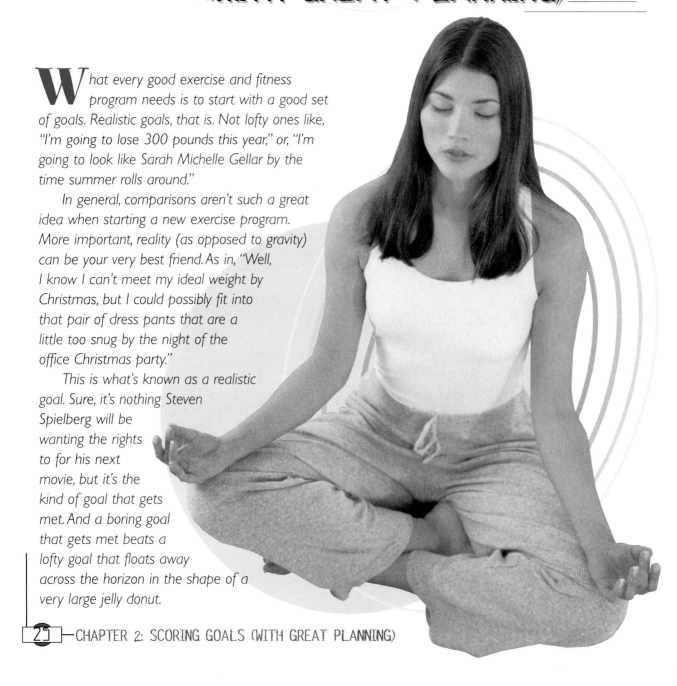

What every good exercise and fitness program needs is to start with a good set of goals. Realistic goals, that is. Not lofty ones like, "I'm going to lose 300 pounds this year," or, "I'm going to look like Sarah Michelle Gellar by the time summer rolls around."

In general, comparisons aren't such a great idea when starting a new exercise program. More important, reality (as opposed to gravity) can be your very best friend. As in, "Well, I know I can't meet my ideal weight by Christmas, but I could possibly fit into that pair of dress pants that are a little too snug by the night of the office Christmas party."

This is what's known as a realistic goal. Sure, it's nothing Steven Spielberg will be wanting the rights to for his next movie, but it's the kind of goal that gets met. And a boring goal that gets met beats a lofty goal that floats away across the horizon in the shape of a very large jelly donut.

REALISTIC NEXT-PECTATIONS, OR: A NEW BE-THIN-ING

Congratulations! You have realized that perhaps it is time to shape up. You've done a little evaluating and the results are less than positive. Unfortunately, appreciating that you need to exercise is only the first step on a very long, arduous, uphill, uneven road, especially because, on average, Americans as they age gain five pounds per decade. There are some questions worth starting with: How much weight do you need to lose, if any? Remember that body fat percentage is more important than poundage. But the scale is still a measure most people use. How will you lose the weight, and keep it off? How long will it take to lose the weight?

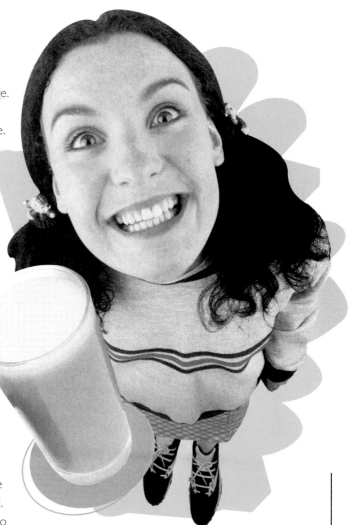

You have seen commercials for a diet product, and the client is "so happy" and has "so much energy" and it all happened with delightful speed and was "so easy!" If you read the fine print, you will see the words "Results not typical." You want to believe, but you know it's not realistic to imagine yourself drinking a runny milkshake twice a day for the rest of your life. Even with four whole flavors! Plus there's the impossible: "And I've kept it off for two years!" Most humans need variety; the more stringent the diet, the less likely you are to stick to it forever, in which case, why bother? Dramatic, rapid results rarely last.

So here's the scoop: By learning how to eat properly and exercise your body, you can expect to lose about a half a pound a week. Sometimes this rate varies, but on average, these realistic results are typical. The slower your weight loss, the more likely you are to adapt to your new habits and train yourself to maintain low body fat long term.

Start thinking about this bumpy road as though it will take more than two years to travel the length. You must allow for the disturbances, hardships, and obstacles you might encounter during any long journey. At the end is the reward for your expedition: a healthy, strong body.

Muscle Myth: *You have to be athletic to exercise.*
Triceps Truth: *Many types of exercise do not require any special athletic abilities. If you can walk or ride a stationary bike without falling off, you are athletic enough to become fit.*

Your function in this capacity is not to judge your body with your own unreliable perceptions; it is to discover the healthiest biological weight for your height and body type, and to begin to change unhurriedly to that end. The advice in these chapters will help guide you.

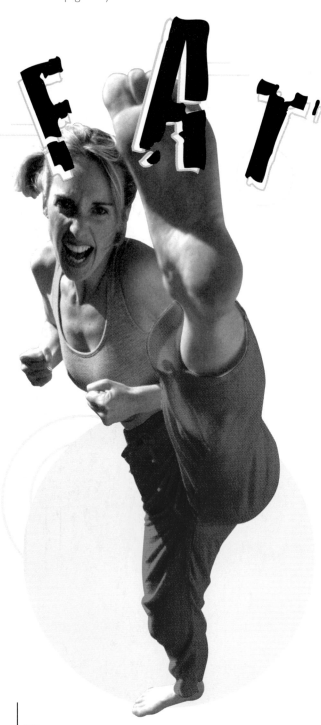

To lose weight, you must burn more calories than you take in, forcing the body to fall back on stored energy, fat, and burn that up instead. This is a perfectly realistic biological system that works very efficiently.

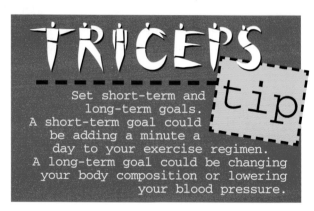

This is remarkably difficult to achieve when the calorie fires are barely stoked. You must fan the flames a little; take a walk in the park. You must walk, swim, bike, run, row, skate, or climb for 30 minutes a day every day, five or six days a week. Just move around for 30 minutes, will you? That's a realistic goal, and don't look beyond it.

Concentrate on the now, and how your body is responding to this attention. The stronger you become, the higher you can raise your goals. You will not lose weight without moving your limbs on a consistent basis, no matter what that diet ad says.

Of course, you've been living on fast food, little sleep, and no exercise for years; old habits die extremely hard. Chastising yourself for skipping a workout is poisonous to motivation. It leads to more skipped workouts, because you begin to suspect that you are not resilient enough for this life change. If you can't face your 30 minutes today, walk around the block, bike to the end of the street, or skip rope during the commercials of your favorite TV show. These are realistic alternatives to omitting your daily activity; you may find that once you get to the end of your street, the end of the next street looks mighty inviting, except for that Rotweiller. Remember, you are in charge here. All-or-nothing just isn't realistic. Sorry.

TRICEPS tip

Set short-term and long-term goals. A short-term goal could be adding a minute a day to your exercise regimen. A long-term goal could be changing your body composition or lowering your blood pressure.

GOAL FOR IT!
OR: PHYSIQUE POINTERS

The world is full of people with good intentions: Pauly Shore. Tony Soprano. You. Sure, it's easy to get psyched up about something and say you are totally committed. However, once the elation dies down and the work part starts, some of you might wane a little in the follow-through department. Yes, you, with the pizza in one hand and a beer in the other.

Once you have a plan, scratch that, a realistic plan, you are halfway to your goal. And once you apply the reality and objectivity of a calendar, and a few handy other tools, you're more than halfway there before you even break a sweat.

EVALUATION STATION

The first step is to evaluate your current health status and physical ability. For instance, do you play a sport on the weekend or do you huff and puff just walking from your car to your front door? It is always a good idea to check with your doctor before starting any new fitness program, especially if you haven't exercised in some time or you have health or physical issues. This may seem unnecessary, but the whole point of starting a fitness program is to improve your health, not to diminish it. Your doctor may also be very helpful in suggesting exercises and diets that will boost your efforts and give you faster results.

METABOLIC MAP

Make a goal map. Actually write down specifically what you want to achieve and by when you want to achieve it. For example, I want to: 1) Lose 10 pounds,

2) Tone my upper body, and 3) Be able to run eight miles in 50 minutes by the end of six weeks. Then, evaluate your goals and determine if they are realistic. Be honest. If the only running you have ever done is to the store to buy a gallon of ice cream, you may need a little more time. However, if you already run or work out on a semi-regular basis, these goals are reasonable and realistic. It is easy to get caught up in the excitement and make huge expectations and demands of yourself. Do not set yourself up for failure.

The next step is to map out the path to your goal. This part can be tricky, especially if you do not have a fitness background. If you are a member of a gym, consult a trainer. Regardless of your fitness goals, a balanced fitness program includes aerobic exercise at least three times per week for at least 20 to 30 minutes, in addition to any needed weight or strength training to tone specific areas. Further, a sensible and balanced diet should also be recommended. However, someone who wants to become a body builder would not take the same advice as a person who simply wants to shed 10 pounds and tone up. It is important to tie in the goal with the method to achieve it. For instance, you

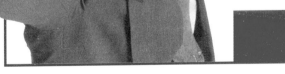

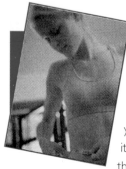

might decide that you need to run three times per week for 30 minutes, in addition to 20 minutes of free weights for your upper body on alternate days. Depending on your goal and current physical status, it may be necessary to set lower goals that lead to your ultimate goal. If this is the case, map out a skeletal outline of what you want to achieve. For instance:

Goal 1: Walk for 30 minutes four times per week, lose 10 pounds within six weeks.

Goal 2: Walk for 30 minutes two times per week and jog for 30 minutes two times per week, lose 10 pounds within six weeks.

Goal 3: Jog for 30 minutes four times per week, lose 10 pounds within six weeks.

Ultimate Goal: Jog for 40 minutes four times per week, lose a total of 20 pounds within 36 weeks.

Once you reach one of your smaller goals, reevaluate your next goal to determine if it is too difficult or too easy. Adjust your next goal's activity and timeline as needed. Once you have a set plan, it is easier to stay focused. You are not floundering with thoughts of what to do on any given day. You know exactly what you need to do, thus safeguarding yourself against being distracted.

Deltoid DIARY

"Spring Break Slim"

Every college girl has the same thought process when it's time to go back to school. "When I get back to campus, I am going to work out every day and then wow everyone when I go back home for Thanksgiving."

But, of course, when Thanksgiving rolls around and you're still hiding your flabby butt with a shirt tied around your waist, you say, "After Thanksgiving, I'm definitely going to the gym every day and by the time it's Christmas, they're not going to believe how good I look."

Then comes the usual turkey leftovers, slices of pie, and rationalizations like, "I don't have time to go running, I have to study for finals and then hit that keg party!" or "Oh, what's another month, I'll just work out at home over Christmas break."

But we all know how that song goes too.

Motivation is definitely hard to find, especially with no goal

TRICEPS tip

Mowing the lawn is not only useful, it's healthful. Use the push mower for 30 to 60 minutes of grass cutting for a great way to shape up that, er, grass.

in sight and no one to help you get there. That's why when it came time for my spring break in Florida last semester, I pushed aside all the pathetic excuses I was clinging to and decided to take action. The first step was to set a goal. Now, how realistic is it to set your 2-week goal at losing 25 pounds? Instead of creating an impossible fitness goal, I decided that I had exactly one month before my spring break and in that month I was going to pay extra attention to what I was eating, cut down on fatty foods, not eat past 6 p.m., and exercise every day. All I wanted was to not be embarrassed in front of everyone in my bikini.

So, I had the goal, but no moral support. That's where my friend came in. We set up a buddy system. We would e-mail each other every morning, through the day, and at night. I would send her articles and tips I read on health and fitness Web sites, and she would send me motivational words to keep me going.

Whenever one of us was feeling down, fat, or just plain lazy, the other one would boost her up with motivating words ("Off your ass!"), a humorous scenario (like picturing yourself in a bikini with a balloon of a stomach—which isn't actually that funny!), or a threat like, "Do you really want to eat that candy bar? Just think what that chocolate will look like on your thighs!"

The month progressed, and something unusual happened: I began to lose weight! My jeans fit better, I could fit into my skinny roommate's pants, and I had the self-confidence of a supermodel! It was then that I realized starving yourself and getting down about it is not going to shed those pounds any faster. The key is to set a realistic goal and have someone there to help you keep your spirits up. By the time I bared my bod on the beach, my saddlebags and wide butt were under control.

Okay, I didn't look like Elle MacPherson by any means, but I was healthy and happy. The plan turned out to be a good one. And if it can work for me, it can work for anyone.

CALENDAR GIRL (OR GUY): PENCIL YOURSELF THIN!

To help you reach your goals, a calendar is one of the most useful tools in the house. If you have decided to start a new fitness program or find yourself struggling with the one you already have, implementing a calendar system can be helpful in many ways. It centers and gives focus, provides a tool for motivation, makes it easier to evaluate your progress, and helps illustrate your program's strengths and weaknesses. And it doesn't take very long to do.

Starting a new fitness program can feel like walking into a dark, endless tunnel; a calendar system can be a way of determining where you are

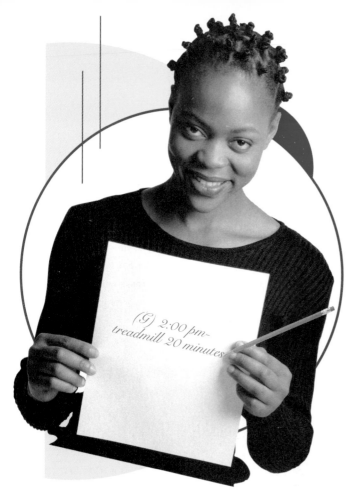

(G) 2:00 pm-
treadmill 20 minutes

So, make exercising a priority by giving it a specific time in your day. Also, write down how you are going to exercise. Be sure to allow ample time for the type of exercise you choose. Do not give yourself 30 minutes to exercise and expect yourself to be able to run 10 miles and do upper body weight training. A sample entry would be:

(G) 2:00 p.m. – treadmill 20 minutes, upper body weights

Then, go back and underneath write down what you actually did. For example,

(G) 2:00 p.m. – treadmill 20 minutes, upper body weights

(A) 2:30 p.m. – treadmill 20 minutes, no weights

Note: You can either write down your "goal" workout and your "actual" workout in different colored pencils, or come up with another way to distinguish them. For example, use (G) and (A), as in the example above.

This way, you can compare what your goal was with what you actually achieved. You will quickly be able to determine if you are expecting too much or too little from yourself, not scheduling enough time for your workout, or even if you are working out at the wrong time of day.

If you did not work out on a scheduled day, be sure to note that also. It only takes a minute to write down the information. Make it a part of the workout. Even if you miss a day of exercising, you still feel connected to your program. Also, if you are keeping track of your weight or measurements, choose a weigh-in or measurement day and write down your goal. Then, write down what your actual weight and/or measurements are on that day.

and what that dimply thing on your thigh might be. The calendar system will organize and focus your time and goals. For example, if you expect to lose 12 pounds in six weeks, write down your desired weight six weeks from the day you start. If your fitness goal is a major change, break it down into smaller steps. This will keep you motivated as you reach your smaller goals.

Furthermore, it will make the goal seem more attainable, as you are tackling it in pieces instead of in one big bite. Write down all of your goals and their timelines. Be sure to do this in pencil in case you need to revise your goals. Nothing is etched in stone.

The next step is to set your exercise time.

Schedule time with yourself to work out. Pencil in your exercise time so that you know exactly when you are expected to do it. This will keep you focused, as you know exactly when you will be working out. It will also keep you from putting it off during the day. You will not just say to yourself, "I need to work out today." You will know exactly when.

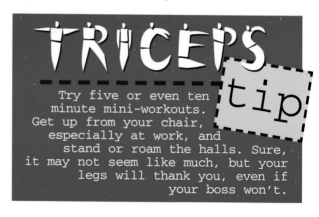

TRICEPS tip

Try five or even ten minute mini-workouts. Get up from your chair, especially at work, and stand or roam the halls. Sure, it may not seem like much, but your legs will thank you, even if your boss won't.

A calendar is also a good way to keep track of your dietary intake, if your program includes closely monitoring your diet. An example entry for this is:

June 7th – Breakfast – 10,500 calories, 400g fat, 12g protein, 10g carbohydrates. (Hey, 200 strips of bacon might be good for you.)

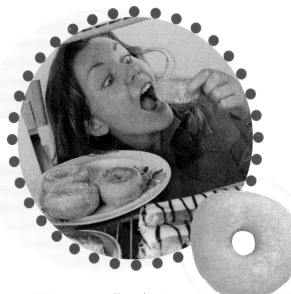

This may seem like a lot to keep track of, but once you get into the habit, it becomes second nature. Take one minute while you are eating to write down what you ate. This is a lot more effective than trying to remember exactly what you ate on any given day. It also eliminates the "snack amnesia" that we all experience while following an exercise program. It can be as detailed as you need it to be. If you just want to keep track of your calories or fat grams, that's fine too.

With your program goals and actual performance written down in front of you, at a glance you will be able to evaluate your program, your progress, your goals, and your program's strengths and weaknesses.

For instance, if you are not losing weight as quickly as you would like, maybe you need to add more aerobics to your program. If you are having difficulty meeting your scheduled workouts or are skipping them altogether, you will be able to determine if your

scheduling needs to be adjusted. If you often feel too tired to work out, try changing your workout time to another time of the day when your energy level is higher. If you are feeling bored with your exercise routine or have reached a plateau, you may decide it is time to try a different sport or exercise. The key is to evaluate yourself and your program on a regular basis. Do not let yourself fall into a rut.

Another advantage of having a calendar system is motivation. Seeing all of the work you have done and all of the goals you have reached will only inspire you to continue. The sense of accomplishment will motivate you to keep going. It also serves to make you accountable. You will have a written statement of your dedication or slacking. It is very disturbing to see unmet appointments and missed goals. You will feel pressure to fulfill the guidelines and goals you have set for yourself.

If you were to keep this information solely in your head, there would be no way to accurately evaluate how you are doing. This way you are in control.

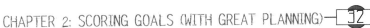

DEADLINE DISTRACTION, OR: (RAT) RACE
AGAINST TIME

Few of us want to wait forever for that perfect body to arrive. Most of us would prefer muscle tone and leaner limbs to appear overnight, preferably while we were still sleeping. Unfortunately, Mother Nature wasn't so kind. And, while that size six dress you've been dying to fit into can stay in the back of the closet for a while, with the proper attitude, a lot of hard work, and a realistic deadline, that body you've always wanted is well within reach. Here's how.

EXERCISING (GOOD JUDGMENT)

Be sure that you choose an exercise program that you enjoy. Exercising won't always be fun or be the activity you want to be doing at that exact moment, but if you hate what you are doing, you won't do it for very long. If you love sports, try incorporating sports into the aerobic part of your program. If you really love the outdoors, try bike riding, inline skating, or surfing. If your program begins to feel stale, try another exercise activity to spice it up.

Don't let yourself get bored. Try a different aerobics video or change your jogging route. Changing your program may also become necessary as the seasons change. Don't let inclement weather or seasonal obligations be your "excuse" not to exercise. Plan ahead. Find something else to do when situations don't permit a regular workout.

"Don't stay in bed—unless you can make money in bed."

—George Burns

THE BUDDY SYSTEM

Another good way to stay focused is to exercise with a partner. A partner can make your program more fun and help make you more accountable. You will have to answer to someone other than yourself. A partner can also assist you with proper exercise form and technique. When you are feeling less motivated, your partner can be there to push you through your distractions.

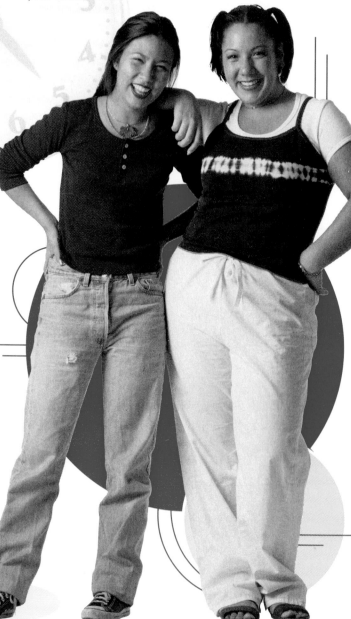

TRICEPS tip

Walk when you can. Park a mile from work. Walk back to the car at lunch. Park an extra block from your destination or at the rear of the parking lot. Look for the longest, rather than the shortest, route and make it a habit rather than just a Monday morning fluke.

TONING UP TOOLBOX

As mentioned before, a calendar is an excellent tool for avoiding distractions. Make appointments with yourself to workout. Write down specifically when and how you want to exercise. Another excellent tool is visualization. Every day visualize yourself achieving your goal. Visualize yourself working toward your goal. When you feel distracted or like you do not really want to follow your program that day, stop and visualize your goals to motivate yourself: See the muscles growing and toning. See the fat actually melting off your body.

REWARD SYSTEM

Also, try setting up a reward system for yourself. For instance, if you follow your program for an entire week, you get to buy yourself something special. If you achieve your goal weight, allow yourself to buy a special outfit. Caveat: Never have food as a reward. Do not set yourself up for a fall. Food is a huge distraction. It is so easy to fall prey to its alluring comfort. Nothing goes to one's head like chocolate. (Or whipped cream, or pasta, or donuts, or...) The reward should be a complement to your fitness program, not a distraction or deterrent.

DETOURS, NOT DOWNFALLS

When mapping out a course to your goal, be sure to prepare for detours. Setbacks should be expected, especially if this is your first attempt at a regimented fitness program. Do not allow a detour to derail you. It is very easy to give up after a setback, but don't. The first step is to forgive yourself. It's in the past; just leave it there and move on. Next, determine if the setback has changed your timeline. For instance, if you have not worked out for a couple of weeks, you may need to adjust your timeline to accommodate for the time lost and the recovery time.

The same holds true for bingeing. If you just ate a piece of cake, your goal probably won't be in jeopardy. However, if you ate an entire cake every day for a

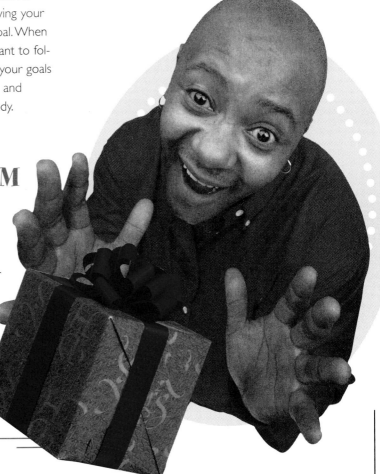

week, you just may have to rework your timeline. The key is not to feel badly about having to change your goal date, but rather to feel pride in your resolve to try again. Look at the positive and see a person determined to reach his or her goal.

POSITIVE ENERGY

The most important components in any endeavor are desire and action. If you want it badly enough and are willing to work for it, you will reach your goals. Be positive and be willing. When beginning a new fitness program, you need to see it as changing your lifestyle. It will not always be fun and you will not always want to adhere to the plan, so you have to make it important enough to stave off the urge to be distracted by other things. Exercising needs to be more important than watching TV or surfing the Net.

Evaluate where you are and where you want to be. Map out exactly the path to your goals and don't let anything, even setbacks, distract you.

JUST SCREW IT, OR: EXERCISING EXCUSES

You have the shoes. You have the outfit. And you have the excuses why they should remain in a pile on the bedroom floor. Excuses, excuses—they are the vehicle to failure. Either you can drive that vehicle on the road to cottage cheese thighs or you can turn around and cruise the other way. Here are the top five excuses for not exercising and their counterpositions:

Excuse #1: "I'll work out tomorrow."

Here is a tip: Tomorrow means never. If you often find yourself too tired to exercise, change the time of day you exercise. For instance, if you are a morning person, you should exercise in the morning. Most people can exercise if they are tired on any given day.

However, if they tried to do that every day, they would give up. Find your "zone" time. There are 24-hour gyms all over the place. People also overlook the lunch hour. This is a great time to exercise. You do not have to be at a gym to get a good workout. Walking at a good pace for 30 minutes will

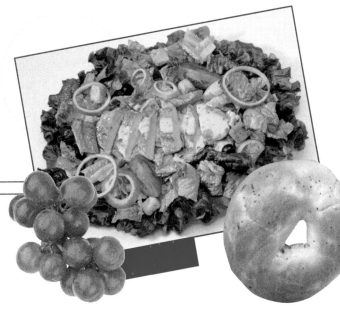

Excuse #2: "I do not feel like it today."

So what? You will not make it to any of your goals if you do not have the discipline to do what needs to be done, even when you do not feel like doing it. Find ways to motivate yourself. Put inspirational pictures on your refrigerator or bathroom mirror. Either these pictures can be of a body type you are shooting for, or of a body type you are desperately trying to avoid. Just put them up where you will see them often. Another way to motivate yourself is to tell several people about your program. It is very difficult to slack off when you are accountable.

Try hooking up with an exercise partner. You two can motivate each other when the "lazies" hit. If you really want to get motivated, go to a store and try on bathing suits or stand in front of a mirror naked.

All joking aside, if your improvement areas are going to be with you, they might as well be useful. Do not obsess about them, just use them.

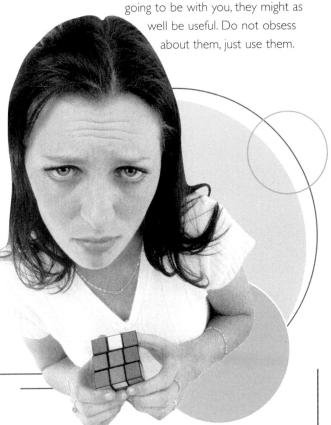

do wonders. You can supplement that with weight training before or after work.

Breaking up your workout is fine. Just make sure that you do your aerobics in blocks of at least 15 to 30 minutes. Exercising at lunch will give you a great lift and help you get through the rest of your day. While your coworkers are feeling tired and weighed down by their heavy lunches, you will feel invigorated. Do not skip your meal; just eat something quick and light.

Other contributors to feeling tired are either eating too much or eating too little. An ideal balanced diet includes protein, carbohydrates, and yes, fat. Further, one should eat five meals per day, not three. By eating five meals, you never get too hungry, so the urge to pig out is kept at bay. Fruit smoothies, chopped fruits and vegetables, low fat–high fiber muffins, cottage cheese, bagels, salads, chicken breasts, and rice are just a few quick and light meal ideas. Although you want to have light meals, they need to be nutritious. One of your meals should not be a candy bar and soda.

Further, resist the urge to skip meals. This will only sabotage your efforts. You will lose muscle mass while storing your existing fat and contributing to your lethargy. When battling the "I am too tired" excuse, look at when you are working out and how well you are eating. Make any needed scheduling and menu changes and get back to work!

Remember why you decided to start exercising in the first place.

Look at your negative areas and visualize them turning positive. Actually see your body morph into the way you want it. Tap into the excitement you will feel once you have reached your goals, and then get going. Make a deal with yourself. Start exercising, and if in 15 minutes you still want to quit, then stop. Nine times out of ten, you will keep going.

Nothing worth having is easy. Exercise is hard work. However, you must weigh that hard work against how bad you will feel when you do not reach your goals. Think it through. It is easy to blow off your program if you do not think about what it really means to do so. It is not just going home and sitting on the couch. It is one less step you have taken toward a goal that is important to you. It is one more day away from the pride in a job well done. It is one more time you let yourself down.

Excuse #3: "I travel too much to exercise."

If you are not careful, you will have to start buying two seats on the airplane. Following an exercise program while being a frequent traveler takes only a little bit of planning. When making hotel reservations, try to find one with gym facilities. Often, if a hotel does not have on-site facilities, the management will have an agreement with a nearby gym to allow guests complimentary access.

If a gym is not available, convenient, or your cup of tea, you can try jogging or walking. Weather and environment permitting, this is a great way to exercise. Further, running shoes, shorts, and a T-shirt are easy to pack. However, if you happen to be staying in a demilitarized zone in the middle of a snowstorm, you can always run or walk the inside stairwells. Do not rule out working out in your room. Most hotels provide VCRs. There are multitudes of exercise videos available, everything from

yoga to kick boxing. You can even rent them from a video store to try them out before you use them.

If videos are not your thing, you can concentrate on strength exercises. It does not take a lot of room to do sit-ups, push-ups, squats, lunges, etc. You can even get weights that you fill with water and empty when finished. You may even have room on a balcony or hallway to jump rope. The old cliché is true: "Where there's a will, there's a way."

Excuse #4: "I cannot exercise because my friends are in the way."

These people blocking your exercise regimen can be your biggest cheerleaders. The trick is to get them involved. You may have to revamp how you exercise. However, if you cannot do your current program anyway, what is the point? Try doing an exercise video they can do, too. They can also do strength exercises like sit-ups and squats next to you.

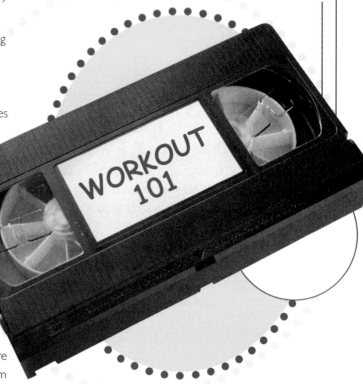

Excuse #5:
"I am too sick/sore/injured to work out."

This may be the only valid excuse to skip exercising. If you are ill, your body is working hard to fight off your illness. It will not be as effective or efficient. Further, exercising may deplete your body's resources and prolong the illness. Consult your physician before working out. If you are experiencing a minor illness, wait until your strength has returned before starting back. Do not push it your first time back. Take it slowly and see how you feel. If you work out at a gym, be sure you are no longer contagious. Nobody else wants to pick up your illness via your coughing or sweat.

Sore muscles should also be heeded. You should give your muscles 24 to 48 hours of rest between workouts. So, if you worked your upper body one day, do your lower body the next day. It is the tearing down of the muscles during the exercise and the rebuilding during the rest period that builds bigger and stronger muscles. So, if you find yourself walking like a cowboy fresh off a cattle drive, or you have to swing your arms to get them up on your desk, take a 24-hour break. Use that time to rework your program to accommodate necessary rest periods.

Injuries are another story. Pushing an injury is one of the most counterproductive things you can do. If you have seen or are continuing to see a doctor for the injury, ask him/her when you can start back. Starting too soon or too rigorously will only prolong the injury and your down time. Further, ask your doctor if you can exercise the rest of your body, or if you can do a different type of exercise. For instance, if you have injured your foot, maybe you can still do sitting upper body weights or swim in a pool. Make sure to follow your doctor's advice to avoid prolonging the injury.

If your injury is not serious enough to see a doctor, rest it until it does not hurt anymore. If possible, you should try working other parts of your body or doing a different type of exercise. When you begin to exercise the healed area, be sure to start slowly. If you feel a twinge, back off, rest a bit longer, and try later. The whole point of a fitness program is to improve your health, not hinder it. Try not to get frustrated. You will get back to your routine and goals much faster if you take care of yourself.

If you do not want to exercise, you will find an excuse not to do it. Ultimately, your desire and discipline will make or break you. If you need a break every now and then, take it. However, if you are not exercising because of roadblocks, be creative and find a way around them. If it is important enough to you, you will.

TO BULK
OR
NOT TO BULK

Weight training can be confusing to any exerciser, whether an amateur or a pro. When you're new to it, you either have fantasies of looking like Linda Hamilton in *Terminator 2* or dreams of finally being able to kick your older brother's ass. The pictures in your head (while pathetic) are great motivators to get you into the gym but, once you're there, you may not know where to start. Should you lift heavy or light? Should you do five reps or 25? Should you do one set or five?

If you're a newbie, just about anything you lift at this point (excluding that cheap beer in your hand) is going to add strength and size to your weak little body.

Later, when you've filled out a bit, you'll have to come up with a program that's going to give you what you want. It all comes down to building lean body mass, and how much you want to have depends on you.

BUILDING YOUR STRENGTH

Now that you've set your goal to look like a *Baywatch* lifeguard, it's time to get to work. If you're a woman and you want to look like Pamela Anderson, go out and get a boob job and then start your strength-training program. You certainly don't want to bulk up like Attila the Hun and, thankfully, most women don't have to worry about that. When it comes to weight training, men and women really are different. Women don't produce as much testosterone as men do and, therefore, most women will never build big hulking muscles, even when following the same routine as a man (unless they're named Chyna).

So, if you're a woman, you can build muscle and

strength without adding too much size. The trick is to keep your repetitions between 12 and 16 and to lift enough weight so that you can complete only the chosen number of repetitions and no more. And make sure your form is perfect. If you're not sure what perfect form is, this would be a great time to introduce yourself to your fitness club staff.

Experts generally recommend two or three sets of each exercise, although you could do more if you're into self-torture. If you are one of the unfortunate few women who tend to bulk up and that's not what you're after, reduce the weight and increase the repetitions.

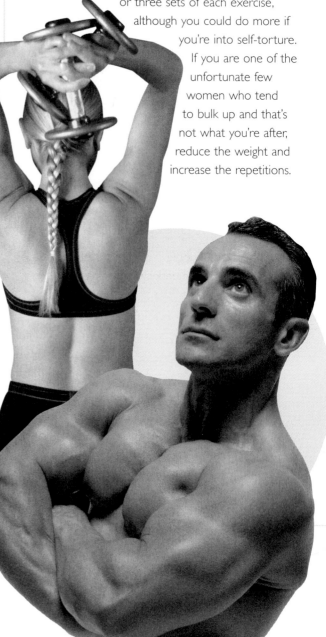

Just don't do more than 20, because you've got better things to do than sit around a gym all day pumping iron.

If you're a man and want to look like a lean, mean fighting machine, use the same rule as above: 12 to 16 reps with the heaviest weight you can handle—with perfect form (no cheatin' boys). Since you're loaded with testosterone, all you have to do is think about lifting a weight and you'll build muscle somewhere. In general, building strength can involve any exercise you want, as long as you're doing it properly and using enough weight and it's an exercise that actually works a muscle group. Making up your own moves is not a good idea. There are tried and true exercises for each muscle of the body and there's a reason everyone does them. Why? Because they work, you moron.

When you're a beginner, you're probably focused on taking care of those pesky weaknesses that have crept up over the years (like the fact that your right arm can curl 25 pounds while your left arm can't even hold a pencil without cramping). Once you've gotten yourself back into proportion, start focusing on the body parts you want to strengthen.

For example, if you want to wow that cute coworker with your flawless shoulders, pick three shoulder exercises that will target each area of your shoulder (like rear deltoid raises, overhead presses, and front raises). Pick a weight for each exercise that will allow you to do twelve repetitions. If you can do more than that, you're cheating and you need to add more weight. In fact, you should add a little more weight to each of your exercises every week or do an extra repetition each time. If you don't keep it challenging, you'll end up in a rut, and no one will ever love you. *Important Note*: Never work the same muscle group two days in a row. They don't like it and will let you know in the form of pain and injury. Let them rest for at least 48 hours before torturing them again.

WHEN SIZE MATTERS

Get your mind out of the gutter, cause we're talking about muscle size here. Um, no not that muscle. When your goal is to make like Arnold, you have to work a lot harder at your routine. If you ever hang around with power lifters or bodybuilders, you'll probably hear things like "max out" or "max power." That's he-man, she-woman talk for taking your muscles to their absolute limit. For the greatest muscle mass increase you have to produce maximum power. Makes you shiver doesn't it? The rule is, you must engage as many of your muscle fibers as possible, and you have to work those aching fibers to the greatest possible intensity. That means taking it to complete and utter failure (a concept you should be familiar with).

What this means is that, instead of doing 12 to 16 reps, you'll pare everything down to four to six repetitions and increase your weight so that, on that last repetition, it takes every ounce of strength, and will take everything you've got (and probably every person in the gym) to get that weight up. Have you ever seen some poor slob on the leg press machine with 700 pounds on each side and wondered why he's screaming and why there are five incredible hulks hovering over him? That's how many people it takes to help that poor bastard finish his last rep. Is it starting to sink in yet?

Not only are you going to have to drastically increase your weight and lower your reps, you're also going to have to do a few more exercises for each muscle group. There's no set rule for how many exercises you should do for each body part. It helps, though, if you know which body part you're working (e.g., the biceps curl is for your biceps muscle—got it?) and how to get at that muscle from several different angles (like the shoulder example from before). You probably want to do at least three exercises for each muscle group, and maybe even as many as five if you're in a sadistic mood.

When it comes to building huge amounts of muscle mass, it's a good idea to plan your workouts with care before going into the gym. As stated above, your muscles need to have time to repair themselves, especially when you're taking them to complete failure. To that end, most bodybuilders split their workouts.

Some work an upper body muscle every day (for example, Monday is chest day, Tuesday is shoulder day, etc.) and then either skip their leg workout (how many bird-legged muscle-heads have you seen?) or combine it with another exercise. Some do all "push" exercises one day, and then "pull" exercises the next. The possibilities are endless, so use your brain or pick the brains of that big scary guy on the bench press. He'll probably be glad to brag about his routine and he'll be sure to give you a spot if you need one.

IMPORTANT THINGS TO REMEMBER

What you should keep in mind is that strength automatically comes when you're building size, but you don't have get big to build strength. It's completely up to you what type of suffering you want to put your body through. Just make sure you're eating enough to fuel your body throughout your workout and, for Pete's sake, get enough sleep, too. Your muscles will thank you and you'll be ready for the (muscle) beach in no time.

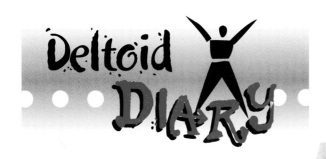

Treadmill Taboo

I'm a bit of a newcomer when it comes to exercising in a gym. All right, we're all friends here, right? Let me be honest then. I'm a bit of a newcomer when it comes to exercising. Period.

My first trip to the meeting place of the muscular was rather enlightening. Apparently, there are some things that are just not acceptable in the workout world. Peeking at another woman's treadmill seems to top the list.

I'm a writer (no need to argue with me here, okay). I like to observe people. I tend to look around, take in my surroundings. And, of course, there's only so long I can stare at my own desperately average body in the giant mirrors before I'm ready to puke.

So while I rhythmically sweated it out to the steady beat of Ricky Martin's latest tripe my wandering eye happened to fall on the digital display of my neighboring treader. Who could help but check out the numbers? She'd been on the machine an impressive twenty-six minutes, but according to her distance she'd only logged in 1.7 miles. And she didn't even have it on an incline. Now, I'm not one to judge, but do the math. She's going to have to pick up the pace a little if she wants to reverse the damage of all those bon bons. Oh jeez, look, she's soared way past her target heart rate. I shook my head.

I guess at some point my eye had officially stopped wandering and began staring. I don't recall the exact moment. This woman apparently does. It's amazing how someone sweating that much can dish out a look that icy. It seems I had committed the ultimate fitness faux pas.

You would think I had rifled through her panties drawer or photographed her in the bathroom stall. I had to have violated her in some awful way to elicit her reaction, 'cause she was mad. Real mad. She slapped her towel down so violently, I nearly lost an eye in the exchange. The sweat soaked fabric now shielded my view of her progress (hers too, I might add). Her eyes had turned beady, her breath heavy. I tried to look away. But surrounded by so many mirrors—she was everywhere!

I shut my eyes, it was useless, my equilibrium was all out of whack. There was a scary moment when I slid off the side of my machine. Ricky Martin's party mix pounded incessantly in my head. My spastically flapping arms knocked over my water bottle. I think I twisted my ankle. I looked up, she was still staring and laughing and staring. She deliberately glanced at my pathetic numbers.

That's it: I hung up the towel, so to speak. Completely disregarding the cool-down mode, I packed up my things. How can anyone be expected to perform next to this psycho. What was the big deal anyway? What's her problem? You can't be working out in public, if you're that guarded, that self-conscious. (Especially in a place with that many mirrors and leotards!)

I ask you, what harm is there in innocently comparing stats? It's not like I'm going to publish that she's eaten a few too many bon bons and can hardly walk a fifteen minute mile. It's not like that at all.

3
EQUIPMENT
CHECK

Despite those glossy, flashy, sexy ads you see on TV every night (and why is it always just after your second helping of dessert?), not all muscle matters take place at a gym. Some improvements can occur right at home. From jump ropes to Bowflex, today's home gyms have a wider variety of oblique offerings than ever before. Walk on a treadmill, ride a stationary bike, heft milk jugs full of cement, whatever. And all in the comfort of your living room, den, or garage.

However, to make sure that all of that high-priced equipment doesn't end up being the most expensive coat hangers you've ever owned, you must take great pains to put yourself into a "gym" state of mind. (Even though you're in a broom closet state of room.)

When building a home gym, however, trust your own good judgment (and our advice), not your TV set. As in, don't buy that combination rowing/stationary cycle/bread maker you see on QVC at 3 a.m. just because you feel guilty about polishing off the last of the butter pecan ice cream minutes earlier.

Consider your personality type, your fitness goals, and last but not least, your budget. You don't want all the weight loss coming from your pocketbook.

GYM VS. GARAGE?
WHERE TO PARK IT!

Now that you've made the commitment to working out, you've got a few decisions to make. On the top of the list is the choice of exactly where you are going to base yourself for your body transformation sessions. Your town has probably got more than one gym. If you live in a metropolis, the Yellow Pages are no doubt full of them. So should you fork out the dough for a membership at one of these establishments? And if so, which one? Should you go sleek and elegant or sweaty and basic?

Maybe you're better off setting up your own gym at home. It would certainly be a whole lot more convenient. And you'd only be paying once for your setup gear, rather than every month at a commercial gym. Would that be the better way to go? What decision will you make?

The success of this whole exercise buzz is going to hinge upon the answers to those questions. So, take your time to get the facts before making a hasty decision. Let's consider the commercial gym first.

TRICEPS tip

Try dancing for a change. Whether alone or with a partner, there are aerobic styles to suit any preference—and heart rate. Who knows, you might just give your nosy neighbor something to really look at for once!

THE FIT FACTORY

Gymnasiums are, in fact, designed as fitness factories. They work on getting people through the door. The minute memberships stop being sold is the minute that revenue starts to stagnate. The large multi-chain gyms have, as a result, become about as personal as a visit to the dentist. Many small independent gyms have, however, realized that their market advantage depends on personal service. Consequently, these gyms often provide a friendlier, less meat market atmosphere. Their equipment may not be as new or as high tech as that found in the bigger, more high profile establishments, but it will be sufficient for your needs. The personal service should easily offset the missing sparkle.

For an annual fee, the gym will provide all of the equipment you'll ever need. But the aforementioned need for bodies to pass through the doors may also mean that you, after spending 10 minutes warming up, find yourself frustratedly cooling down again as you join a queue waiting to use a popular piece of equipment. Factor in the fuel and time you'll be eating up traveling to and from the gym, the fact that you'll be limited to the gym's operating hours, and that you'll be subjected to the stares of hundreds of strangers each time you hit the plates, and the

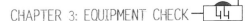

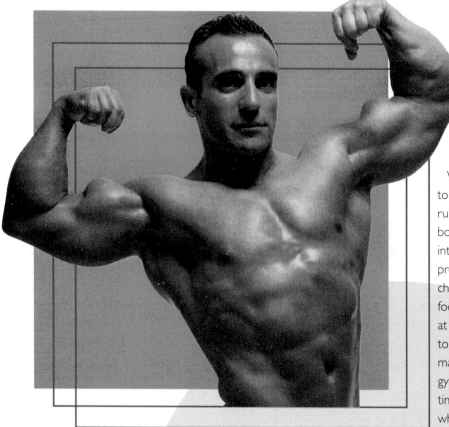

means that you can get a vast range of health related services and advice all under one roof.

So, if you decide to throw in your lot with a commercial gym, what should you look for? Well, first and foremost you need to feel comfortable in the place. If rubbing shoulders with 230 pound bodybuilders leaves you slightly intimidated, the local Gold's is probably not going to be your first choice. Are you able to keep your focus off the inevitable babe line up at the weight stations? If this is going to be a distraction (be honest) you may be better off at a single sex gym. Take a tour of the gym at the time you intend to work out to see what goes on when you're going to be there. There's a big difference in activity at gyms between 2 p.m. and, say, 5 p.m.

comforts of the home gym may sound quite appealing.

Make no mistake, however: Commercial gyms do have several distinct advantages. Consider the following:

• Qualified instructors should be on hand to help you get your technique right and to guide you along on a weight training, aerobic, and nutritional program that will have you safely progressing toward your goals.

• The extra motivation of the gym environment may well make it easier for you to stay on track with your fitness quest.

• The very act of forking out for a membership is an incentive to make those dollars count by sticking with your initial commitment.

• You should have all of the equipment available that you need (so long as you avoid peak times).

• Many gyms are now holistic in their approach. This

If you can, choose a gym that is not too far from your home. If it's within comfortable walking distance that's great. Studies show that the farther a person has to go to get to the gym, the less likely he is to go. So, give yourself the edge by choosing a gym that is not too far out of the way. The ideal, of course, would be if the gym were located along your route between work and home.

Check out the gym staff. They should all be certified by the likes of the American Council on Exercise or the American College of Sports Medicine, as well as being trained in CPR and first aid, in the event you simultaneously have a heart attack and drop a five-pound barbell on your toe after seeing the woman on a nearby mat contort herself in a way you are sure is not authorized in the Bible.

Find out how many trainers are on at peak times and, as you tour the gym, observe whether they are actually helping the members. If they're chatting together about last night's episode of *Friends* while some overweight newbie is slowly asphyxiating himself under the weight of a bench press bar, that is a sure sign that you're not going to get the personal attention you deserve. Give the place a miss.

Look for a gym that offers a monthly payment as opposed to an annual one. This will work out to be a little more expensive, but you won't be tied down if circumstances change. Gyms thrive off people who pay for a year and end up coming for only a couple of weeks. If for any reason you have to stop going, at least you won't be losing a fortune. Make sure you check the fine print on your gym contract, too. Are there hidden costs—like for use of the pool or sauna? Make sure you know exactly what you're in for before you commit.

THE GARAGE GYM

Maybe you've decided you'd be better off with your own personalized workout studio at home. Is this really the best option? Maybe, but you've got to have the discipline to make it work. If you feel that you've got the mental grunt to pull it off, there are some real advantages to working out at home. Of course, your workouts are on tap—you can do them whenever you want. You don't have to compete with a roomful of broad shouldered behemoths for the equipment and you're not forking out dead money for a membership. Still, the big worry is motivation. This nation is littered with costly home fitness gear that is rusting away in closets or acting as very uneconomical clothes horses. To make sure that your home fitness program doesn't

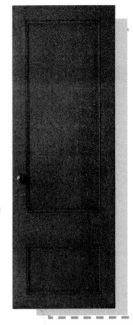

go to the pack, consider the following motivation enhancers:

- Get yourself a workout buddy. When you've got someone else relying on you, it's a lot harder to wimp out.

- Set a workout schedule that allows you to get your workout done early. You're going to have to get a grip on mind over mattress syndrome, but early morning workouts allow you to get it out of the way. You're less likely to have appointments or distractions at 6 a.m.

- Get properly set up. You don't want to be frustrated with dumbbells that collapse on you or cables that disengage. Keep yourself on track by investing in decent equipment.

- Allow a permanent space for your workout gear. If you have to move the car, pull out the lawn mower, and shift the kids' bikes to get at the bench press, you're going to have less enthusiasm for the workout to follow. So, make your workout as accessible as possible.

TREADMILL TESTIMONIALS

That all sounds fine, of course, if you happen to be the proud owner of a sprawling 20 room mansion. What about us lesser mortals, though, who are struggling to accommodate our roomies in our already overcrowded living quarters?

Where are we going to find some extra space for the extravagance of a home gym? Well, it's here where a little bit of lateral thinking wouldn't go amiss.

Consider, for instance, what others like yourself have done to build out some exercise space:

Bob from Baltimore didn't have one spare inch of floor space available to accommodate his exercise needs—or so he thought. When he decided to look outside of the square, he realized that there were tons of unused space going to waste. Where? Above his head. Yes, Bob was able to utilize the space available in his attic. Before you haul your weights up there, however, make sure that the attic floor is sufficiently reinforced to prevent any nasty crashes. A barbell through the ceiling isn't going to do much for your home's resale value.

Cindy from Cincinnati was able to coax her handy-man neighbor, Harold, to enclose her carport. This not only saved her 1986 Honda from the elements, it provided some space where Cindy could set up a compact but workable home gym.

Tom from Texas didn't have a carport or an attic. What he did have was a buddy with some extra room at his crib. By sharing the cost of equipment, Tom was not only able to find a home for his workouts but also a workout partner.

So, don't write off the possibility of a home gym because you think you don't have the space. Rather, give your brain a little exercise. Who knows what you'll come up with?

"CRUNCH"-ING THE NUMBERS,
OR: "EXERCISING" GOOD JUDGMENT
WHEN HOME FITNESS SHOPPING

So, it's two in the morning and you still can't sleep, so you go for that pint of Ben & Jerry's in the fridge and work that clicker, trying to find a little true crime on late-night cable. Unfortunately, the folks at Court TV have locked up shop for the night and have turned things over to the folks at Infomercials Are Us. Where there used to be blood, chalk lines, and guts there now lie veggie steamers, luggage sucking vacuum packers, and microwave egg cookers.

And then, just before your last bite of Chunky Monkey, is the answer to your dreams: An exercise machine offering ultimate fitness at the low, low, low price of only $69.95—in 400 easy installments! "Yes!" you whisper to yourself, not wanting to wake the whole house as you scrounge around for a pen and piece of paper to write down the 800 number located somewhere in beautiful Boise.

Sound familiar? Sure it does. We all want to exercise, shape up, slim down, and look better. But we also don't want to go out of our way to do it. So what better answer than the odd piece of home exercise equipment or two? Well, nothing really. That is, if you actually use it. The trouble is, most of those multi-hundred dollar pieces of expensive exercise equipment get sweat on for a day or two, and then slowly subside into the world of expensive artifacts and future garage sale markdowns.

Still, if you'd like to know how to buy

the best exercise equipment, and actually use it, here are a few helpful tips.

TOTALLY!

As you begin shopping, look for equipment that offers a total workout. The best route to overall fitness is one that incorporates a variety of physical

activities as part of a daily routine. Therefore, try to find a machine that offers a workout not only for your heart, but for your upper and lower body as well. Examples are exercise bikes that have moving handrails that provide resistance, rowing machines that work your legs and arms, and those rubber band and weight bench contraptions that convert into "complete" home gyms with exercises such as the bench press or leg curls.

While many of these "all-in-one" gyms can be found, as seen, on late-night or early TV, your best bet is to shop for one locally so that you can actually try it out. With so many varieties, you'll do yourself a great disservice by buying one on impulse just because it was the first one you saw while walking by the phone. After all, such a big monetary and time investment requires a little research first.

Speaking of cost, it's obvious that a piece of equipment that combines exercises for all of your body is expected to take up all of your extra cash. For a few months, anyway. But many times the money is worth it, if you compare it with buying machines for each separate part of your body, well, separately: exercise bike, weight bench, ab cruncher, etc.

However, if you are the type of person who enjoys a brisk walk or morning jog to exercise your leg muscles and get your cardiovascular workout, you might not need an all-in-one machine. Similarly, if you already own a weight bench and a set of free weights, you won't need the upper portion of an all-in-one contraption.

Naturally, it behooves you to sit tight and write a list of needs and, more important, "don't needs," before you invest in any piece of exercise equipment, especially one that will take up most of an entire room. (Not to mention an entire paycheck.)

REALITY BITES

Before investing in an exercise machine, however, remember that you should be doing it for all the right reasons, and none of the wrong ones. For instance, if you're buying it just to keep up with your old college buddies, that's a wrong reason. So is buying one because you have a crush on the UPS man. More important, don't buy an exercise machine because you think it's going to be the answer to all of your health problems. No hunk of metal and foam, rubber band and leg lifts will turn that beer belly into six pack abs if you don't use it, as prescribed, on a regular basis. Continuing to eat your nightly pint(s) of Chunky Monkey, similarly, without using the machine, will not magically cause it to burn calories while you're not looking. Buying an exercise machine is only a part of your regular exercise routine. An integral part, yes, but a part nonetheless. Your commitment, motivation, and determination are parts as well. Parts that, in time, could mean more results than any machine ever could.

BE SKEPTICAL OF
OUTRAGEOUS
CLAIMS

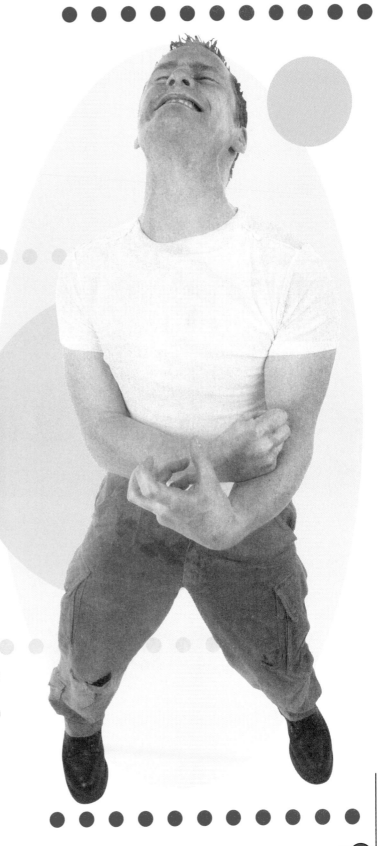

Returning to our example, you're watching yet another infomercial and downing yet another pint of Ben & Jerry's best. You're watching that pocket fisherman commercial for the five hundredth time and, suddenly, a legion of young, hip, gorgeous, fit, good-looking wannabe stars and starlets (minus the talent) start mouthing off about a particular exercise equipment with their "true" stories and "personal" testimonials.

Can you believe them? Maybe. They must be doing something right, after all. But, just as easily, that something could be working out for six hours a day with a personal trainer. So, are they lying? Probably not. Maybe they do use the machine in question. Once or twice a week, to keep from actually "lying," that is.

More important, what do their claims have to do with you? Perhaps you're a different body type than those shown in the commercial. Maybe you're too tall or too short for the machine in question. Don't be fooled by white teeth and firm tummies into buying a machine you won't use because it's not comfortable, simple, or even practical.

Remember: Shaping up is hard to do. Ads that promise "easy" or "effortless" results are false. And many ads that make big claims about the number of calories you'll burn also may be faulty. Can you see through outrageous claims? Exercising regularly can help you shape up. But some companies claim that you can get results by using their equipment for three or four minutes a day, three times a week. Sounds fabulous, right? But realistic? Not likely.

"CRUNCH"-ING THE NUMBERS

Whether you're buying your home exercise equipment in the store or over the phone or Internet, get the total cost of the product before you buy. Remember, the total cost includes sales tax, shipping and handling, delivery, and possibly set-up fees. Machines that advertise for $49.95 monthly may seem to compete with those costly gym fees, but if an asterisk follows the price, that means there may be hidden fees that drive the monthly cost up to sixty or even seventy dollars.

Also, get the details on warranties, guarantees, and return policies. Especially if you're buying over the phone or the Web. Check out the company's customer service and support, too, in case you need replacement parts. Try any toll-free numbers to see if they really work!

GOAL!

What are your goals? Whether you want to build strength, increase flexibility, improve endurance, or enhance your health, look for a program that meets your personal goals. Remember that the best route to overall fitness and health is one that incorporates a variety of physical activities as part of a daily routine.

THE WANT "ABS"

Occasionally, you can get a great deal on a piece of fitness equipment from a second-hand store, a consignment shop, a yard sale, or the classifieds in your local newspaper. But buy wisely. Items bought second-hand usually aren't returnable and don't have the warranties of new equipment.

MAKE READING AN EXERCISE, TOO

Have you checked the fine print? Look for tip-offs that getting the advertised results requires more than just using the machine. Sometimes the fine print mentions a diet or "program" that must be used in conjunction with the equipment. Even if it doesn't, remember that diet and exercise together are much more effective for weight loss than either diet or exercise alone.

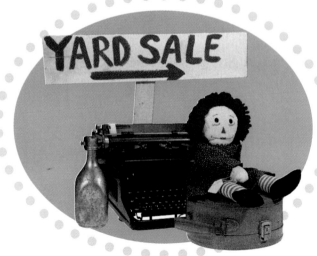

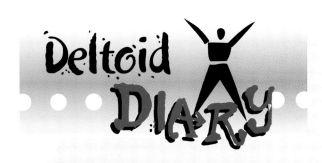

Deltoid DIARY

ME, MYSELF & I, OR: Look Ma, I'm Weightless

Dumbbells, benches, leg presses, abdominal machines, universal gyms—the list goes on. There is so much exercise equipment out there; I would hate to be a beginner looking to purchase the "perfect piece of equipment." Of course, as you might have already figured out, there is no perfect machine, no perfect free weight. It's all a matter of personal preference. Some people like the freedom of standard free weights. Others like the stability of a universal gym.

However, my preference leans in a totally different direction. One that might be called primitive by some, and is considerably overlooked. My favorite machine is no machine at all. My body works as its own

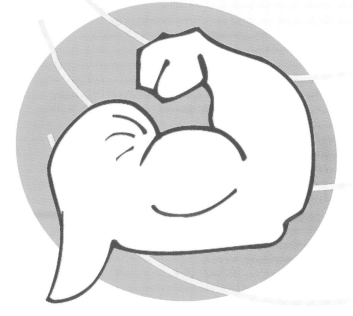

machine and I use myself to strengthen and tone every part of it.

I've used all the different genres of equipment while experimenting with my fitness program. For a while I was hooked on the universal gym. I thought, wow—I can do biceps and lat pull downs, tricep pull downs, cable crosses for my chest, pulls for my back, and crunches with weights all at one machine? What a deal! Of course, when the repetition of walking around a hunk of metal got old, I switched to free weights. I liked the freedom of being able to change up my exercise a lot more. Bicep curls to the front, to the side, tricep push packs, overhead presses, upward rows— fantastic! But, my mind (and my body) got bored with those exercises as well. Boring sucks. It was then that I did something rash. I decided, to heck with them all! I

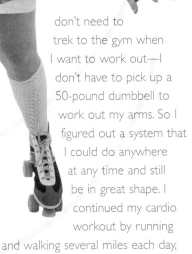

don't need to trek to the gym when I want to work out—I don't have to pick up a 50-pound dumbbell to work out my arms. So I figured out a system that I could do anywhere at any time and still be in great shape. I continued my cardio workout by running and walking several miles each day, but I added in a different part of my new program bit by bit. First I started with push-ups. Yes, push-ups.

Remember those from 8th grade gym class? They're the best workout your arms can get! The set consists of 25 regular, standard push ups (on the toes, not those sissy girl ones from the knees), take a one minute breather and follow it with another set of 25, only this time with your hands in the shape of a triangle. This hand formation works the triceps. After that set, another breather to give those Jell-O arms a break and then back to 25 standard push-ups. Breather, then 25 with the arms bent in on the outsides of your shoulders, in a V-shape. This works the back and shoulders.

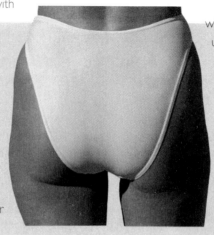

One last breather and finish off with a killer set of 25 standard push-ups. Let me tell you, these babies combined with a regular cardio workout will give you the most cut, muscular arms you've ever seen! And it doesn't take long to see results because you are building muscle and burning fat but not bulking up. Crunches are another perfect exercise. The key to crunches is all in the breathing. Exhale on the way up; inhale on the way down. I don't do a lot of crunches because I focus on my abdominals throughout all of my other exercises. For example, when I am running, I keep my upper body upright, shoulders back, chest up (this also strengthens your shoulders and chest, giving you a leaner upper body), and stomach tight! The deep and excessive breathing you do when you are running gives your abs a workout without you even knowing it. So, keep those abs tight!

Keep the same thing in mind when you are pushing away at those push-ups. So, since I am careful to tighten my abs throughout all my other exercises, I only need to do a few sets of crunches a few times a week to see results. A set of 25 standard upward crunches (hands crossed on the chest for the maximum abdominal workout), 25 to the right, 25 to the left, 25 with the legs in the air, and 25 more standard—and your ab workout is done! Geesh, you've covered your entire upper body without even picking up one weight!

And you could have done this entire workout without leaving your living room! All that is left is your legs and butt. For legs, I prefer lunges and squats. Leg lifts tend not to work the muscle enough to see any actual results, so I do various sets of lunges and squats. You can take a walk around your block doing lunges (you might look kind of silly, but you'll definitely feel the burn) or go back and forth between your right and left legs while watching TV. For squats, do a set of about 40 with the feet facing forward (your legs should be shoulder-width apart) and 40 with the feet facing outward (this gives you an inner thigh workout). Remember to

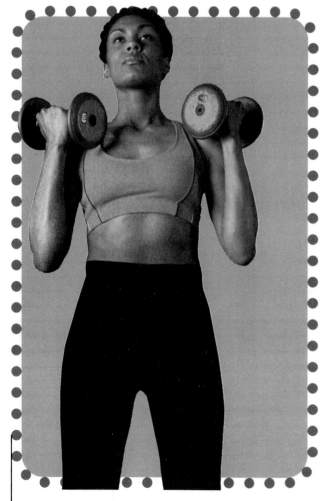

keep those muscles tight, squeeze when you come up, and think "Tight buns!"

People were in shape way before the invention of Soloflex, and you can achieve the same results with your own body! Why do you think Tae-Bo is as popular as it is? No equipment, just use your body. Remember to keep everything tight when you exercise and remember another key—resistance. While running, swing your arms briskly, or when speed walking, punch the air in front of you for added resistance. You'll be amazed with the results. Your body really is the best piece of equipment you can use!

HOME
(HARD) BODIES,
OR: FURNITURE VS.
FITNESS

It's true that gyms provide inspiration, a sense of camaraderie, and a definite atmosphere that is very helpful in motivation. All the newfangled equipment is available for your sweating pleasure: Treadmills, stair machines, and elliptical trainers. Instructors lead spinning classes, Tae-Bo, and Pilates. Hot tubs and saunas complete the experience. Many gyms even house a spa, complete with healthy snacks and massage tables. Many, many people spend hundreds and even thousands of dollars a year in an effort to stay fit—and are successful.

Unless you are in the bothersome predicament of having too much money, you will be happy to know that just as many people spend a few dollars a year and are equally successful at home.

TIPS FOR HOME EQUIPMENT SHOPPING

◎ **Try used sporting goods stores**
◎ **Internet shopping for deals**
◎ **Multiple use machines**
◎ **Online auctions (Check for end-of-the-year sales)**
◎ **Wholesale shopping**
◎ **Split equipment costs with a workout partner**

TRICEPS tip

Recruit a friend. Engaging in physical activities together is a good way to keep a friendship alive and your exercise routine, too.

AEROBIC &
CARDIOVASCULAR
EQUIPMENT

Treadmills, stair machines, and stationary bikes all perform the same function:

They provide calorie-burning, lower-body exercise in the shortest time possible. They are simple, they are affordable, and they are effective.

Unfortunately, they are not the only answer.

If you intend to buy a machine to commit to and rely on for the rest of your life, you are dooming yourself to a lifetime of tedious activity, and one you will be unlikely to stick to. Can you trot into your basement or spare bedroom every single day for all of the years to come, and step onto the same machine, go through the same motions? Imagine, ten years from now, how eager and motivated you will feel as you face the machine (now known as the old ball-and-chain) for about the three thousandth time, assuming you've kept at it this long.

The key, as with everything else in this weight game, is take it easy. Go ahead and buy a machine for rainy days, or for those days when the gym seems so far away, it might as well be on the moon. The machine can be a welcome and comfortable alternative to skipping daily exercise altogether, but it is not realistic to think you can stick to a program devoid of variety. Humans require variety, in all things: music,

reading, lunch meat. That's just the way we are, and we should remember this when considering an exercise program. Before you drop that cash on your dream machine, however, shop around. They differ greatly from brand to brand and model to model. The brands you recognize from the gym are durable, but pricey; the ones decorated with little discount tags are neither. Perhaps you can find a middle ground.

On exercise equipment, shiny objects like readouts, calculations, or measurements often gather dust once their novelty wears off. Gadgets are fun, yes, yes! They are also expensive and often useless, so keep flashy features to a minimum. You should take at least twenty minutes to experiment with the machine and its functions. Would you take a car for a three-minute test drive? Do not settle for a machine with even a few imperfections; less-than-divine is not worth your money. Nagging doubts should be heeded! Ask lots of questions; if the salesperson can't answer them, find someone who can.

Very important is your personal opinion of

the machine. Does it look comfortable? Do you like the color? Is the exercise too demanding for your level of fitness? Unless you're into certain things, a medieval torture device is something you will want to avoid, so make sure this machine fits your personality and

body type. If you have weak knees, don't buy a stair machine, or the instrument of torture will develop into the instrument of holding laundry.

Always remember, this machine is to help you toward your fitness goal; it is not an adversary. If you find yourself approaching exercise machines in general with a degree of hostility, they may not be for you!

WEIGHTS

Free weights are always handy. They are inexpensive and universal; your muscles don't know the difference between a giant can of soup and a two-pound weight. Just as handy is a weight bench with the weights included, also affordable. How much weight do you need? It might be a good idea to test yourself before dropping a fortune on some spectacular, fabulously expensive weight set, so they don't sit abandoned in your basement. Many, many people buy weights and then abandon them, like some unloved toy.

However, this works to your advantage; garage sales, classified ads, and online auctions are an amazing resource for recycled weights. Two each of the two, three, five, eight, ten, twelve, and fifteen-pound weights are pretty much all you need to start a basic set. Now that you have the weights, what do you do with them?

You need to find some routines that challenge each and every muscle group, upper and lower body. (More on the weight routine in Chapter 4.)

VIDEOS

Not all videos are created equal. Rent a few, and if you like them, buy them and pretend they are your personal trainers. Videos are awesome tools for working out at home; they provide structure, cadence, and teach you proper technique. You will need to buy a variety—there's that word again—of videos to keep you motivated and challenged, not always easy at home. Another thing to keep in mind is just how credible you find the instructor. Kathy Smith and Denise Austin are easy to take seriously; their credentials can be confirmed and they've been around a long time.

However, the newest video by the newest supermodel in the newest cut of Lycra leotard defeats the purpose of buying the tape if you're laughing too hard to work out. If you find the person on the video irritating, or if the workout is boring or too complicated, you will not look forward to plugging in your personal trainer day after day! Who would want to anyway, even if the trainer is charismatic? As with exercise machines, you will find it difficult to commit completely to a video in the first place; they must be used in combination with other activities.

Try to set up your workout TV and VCR in a room other than where you usually sit on your ass and stare slack-jawed at the idiot box each night. Remove any distractions, but keep the room pleasant and clean. Even a simple relocation from one room to another can have an effect on your brain: Time to work out!

THE GREAT OUTDOORS

The cheapest, most invigorating place to work out is, of course, your own backyard. A brisk 30-minute walk may be the best thing you can do for your body. Keep your back straight, your head high. Bend your arms to 90 degrees at the elbow and pump them in an arc as you take small, quick steps. Set a destination, like the local bar, or have someone drop you off a half hour from home. The faster you walk and the shorter your strides, the more calories you will burn. This speed walking is actually just as effective, and less harmful to your joints, than running.

Rather than sweating in a stuffy gym, you can also bike, hike, skip rope, inline skate—anything fun that makes you huff and puff for thirty minutes a day. By varying your workouts, and keeping them affordable, you will make it much simpler to find activities you can stick with for the rest of your life. If exercise is a chore, you will never learn to enjoy it, and you may lose interest and stop. The key is to ask yourself: Can I do this very thing for myself every day for the rest of my life? If the answer is yes, you're on the right track. Stay consistent, trust yourself, and trust too that home exercise will give you a healthy body.

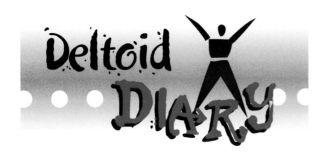

Deltoid Diary

GOING NOWHERE FAST

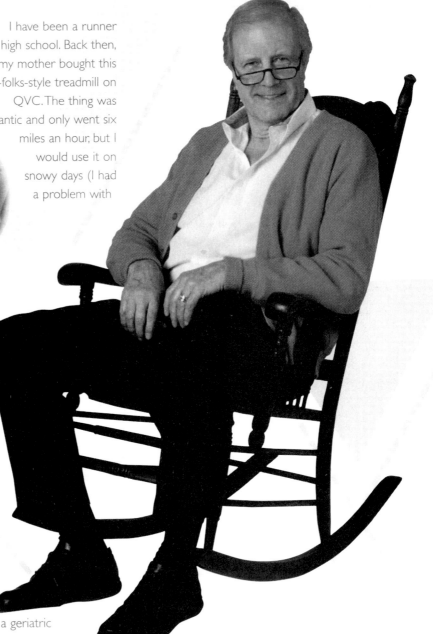

I have been a runner since high school. Back then, my mother bought this old-folks-style treadmill on QVC. The thing was gigantic and only went six miles an hour, but I would use it on snowy days (I had a problem with the cold) and grew sort of addicted to it. Something about its drone, its sluggishness, and the reliability of watching the electronic clock click down the minutes until I was done was soothing.

When I later moved to New York, the sports center where I worked out didn't have treadmills. It had a roof track, at which one could watch the goings-on of New York's Houston Street, and it had a beautiful pool, but no treadmills. Except in a room they called the "Exercise Prescription Room"—which was a geriatric hideout. But, as a runner faced with the bitterness of winter, I had to get into that room for the treadmills. There was no way I was going to dare run outside with the threat of snow, hail—or worse—tourists.

So I did what anyone in my situation would do: I lied. One could get access to this room if one was on a sports team who needed to rehab an injury, so I said I was on the swim team. I'd seen the swimmers around; the pool was usually crowded

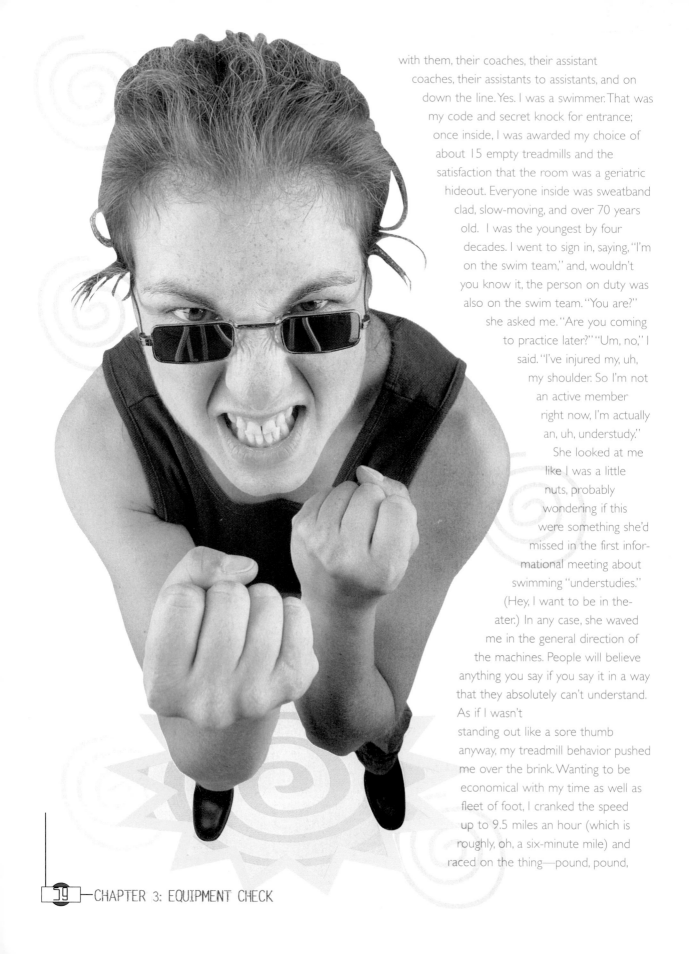

with them, their coaches, their assistant coaches, their assistants to assistants, and on down the line. Yes. I was a swimmer. That was my code and secret knock for entrance; once inside, I was awarded my choice of about 15 empty treadmills and the satisfaction that the room was a geriatric hideout. Everyone inside was sweatband clad, slow-moving, and over 70 years old. I was the youngest by four decades. I went to sign in, saying, "I'm on the swim team," and, wouldn't you know it, the person on duty was also on the swim team. "You are?" she asked me. "Are you coming to practice later?" "Um, no," I said. "I've injured my, uh, my shoulder. So I'm not an active member right now, I'm actually an, uh, understudy." She looked at me like I was a little nuts, probably wondering if this were something she'd missed in the first informational meeting about swimming "understudies." (Hey, I want to be in theater.) In any case, she waved me in the general direction of the machines. People will believe anything you say if you say it in a way that they absolutely can't understand. As if I wasn't standing out like a sore thumb anyway, my treadmill behavior pushed me over the brink. Wanting to be economical with my time as well as fleet of foot, I cranked the speed up to 9.5 miles an hour (which is roughly, oh, a six-minute mile) and raced on the thing—pound, pound,

pound, pound, pound—for three miles. Worse yet, I'd hold on to the sides while running (because, obviously, I'd fall off if I naturally tried to run that fast), practically lifting the treadmill off the ground.

In the middle of the run, overcome with heat, I'd jump to the sides with the treadmill still ripping along and tear off my T-shirt to reveal a fluorescent green, smelly sports bra. Then I'd leap back on and continue my frenzied pace. This got a lot of looks. The administrators of the room tried to throw me out. "What sports team did you say you were on?" they'd ask. Also: "You must stop grabbing the sides of the treadmill like that. You're going to break it. This is an expensive piece of equipment."

"Uh huh," I'd mumble, feeling the eyes from all others in the room on me. "Okay." But I kept doing exactly the same thing every time I came in.

For the most part, though, I felt like the queen of the gym. This bliss continued, and never once did I have to use the roof track in cold weather. This to some extent lessened my interaction with people my own age, but I always thought social run-ins at the gym were kind of strange. God forbid I saw anyone I knew in my weird treadmill revelry. When I did see people I knew, I felt like they'd caught me in this undignified act, as if I'd just been caught sneaking into an AARP strip club. I'd have to explain my "special access" into the old people's exercise room.

As cold weather approached, I noticed that the exercise room was closed. "They're renovating," someone told me. "You can't use it for another eight

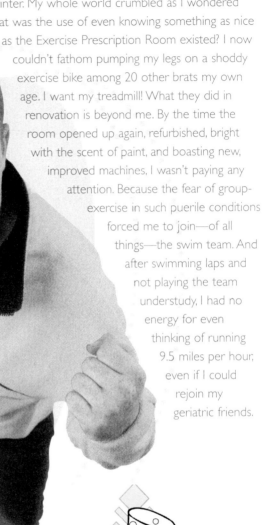

months." I left, wondering how I was going to deal with six loops on the roof track throughout the whole dead of winter. My whole world crumbled as I wondered what was the use of even knowing something as nice as the Exercise Prescription Room existed? I now couldn't fathom pumping my legs on a shoddy exercise bike among 20 other brats my own age. I want my treadmill! What they did in renovation is beyond me. By the time the room opened up again, refurbished, bright with the scent of paint, and boasting new, improved machines, I wasn't paying any attention. Because the fear of group-exercise in such puerile conditions forced me to join—of all things—the swim team. And after swimming laps and not playing the team understudy, I had no energy for even thinking of running 9.5 miles per hour, even if I could rejoin my geriatric friends.

4
GYM
BOUND

So, you've decided to join a gym. Congratulations! Now all that's left to do is lose thirty pounds, buy a whole new workout wardrobe, and plunk down a couple of hundred dollars a month first (plus the initiation fee).

Naturally, gyms or health clubs afford their users a variety of workout equipment, state-of-the-art facilities, and valuable expertise that would be almost impossible to find in, say, your very own garage. You know, the one with the rusty weight set and the 1972 stationary cycle with the grandma-ass seat.

Gyms are also great places to get motivated, with their awesome sound systems, bright lighting, and enthusiastic patrons. Speaking of patrons, gyms are great places to meet other buff buds and bodacious babes like yourself as well.

Before you step inside, however, you'll want to know the basics, such as, where to find a clean towel, what to bring in your gym bag, and where not to direct your eyes in the locker room.

JOINING THE GYM-BOREE, OR: MEMBERSHIP FLEE

It's no secret that health club memberships peak every January. The flabby effects of too many holiday treats hang like ornaments off our winter-fed frames. Thoughts of spring begin to sprout in our minds, and with renewed vigor we commit to "get in shape." But by February, most people who have pledged their Christmas cash to a monthly gym membership are back on their couches "exercising" the remote control. Joining a health club can be a great way to help you maintain a regular exercise program, but it can also turn into an expensive white elephant if you're not careful about choosing a club that meets your particular needs.

WHAT'S IN IT FOR ME?

Begin by thinking seriously about what you want to get out of a club. This doesn't mean scoring hot dates or achieving the perfect body. Be realistic. What time of day will you work out? Figure in at least an hour for traveling to and from the gym, exercising, and showering. What kind of equipment do you need? If you're a lap swimmer and the gym has a wading pool, it ain't gonna work. Do you need childcare while you flex and sweat? Are you more comfortable in a women-only club? Think through your individual needs before you start your search.

Ask for recommendations from your friends and coworkers. Compile a list of clubs and then take each one for a trial run. This is the fun part, and it should be free. Do your homework. Call the Better Business Bureau or Attorney General's office to see if there have been any complaints lodged against the clubs you are considering.

Call each club and ask the salesperson for a trial membership (usually one week). Then do your entire workout during the time of day that you will actually be using the gym. Try the equipment, take a shower, casually ask other members how they like the place. Is it clean and comfortable? Did you have to wait in long lines? Make the most of your trial membership by considering the following points as you go.

YOU CAN'T GET THERE FROM HERE

Sometimes the greatest hurdle to overcome in starting and maintaining a workout schedule is simply getting from Point A to Point B. It's so easy to whine, "It's too far!" and sink further into the couch cushions. So make sure you choose a club that is close to your home or workplace so that you're less likely to skip sessions. You shouldn't have to drive more than 15 minutes to get there. Better yet, pick a place that you'll see driving to and from your home or office. Don't give the "out of sight, out of mind" trick a chance. What if you want to walk, run, or bicycle as part of your workout? Choose a club near a trail or park so you can burn off calories, then retreat to the climate-controlled gym to stretch, shower, and do strength training afterward.

SERVICE IS EVERYTHING

Does the gym offer the services you need? Many health clubs have a variety of aerobic machines, weight-lifting machines, and aerobics classes, but be sure that the machines and classes you prefer are available at the times you'll be using them. Check the club at various hours to see when it's most crowded. The most sophisticated exercise hardware in the world is worthless if you have to wait a half hour to use it. What extra perks does the club offer? Many clubs offer yoga classes, massage therapy, steam rooms, physical therapy, and nutrition counseling. Get the most bang for your buck—and your body!

THE CUSTOMER IS ALWAYS RIGHT

Is the staff helpful and attentive? If you're a beginner, you must get some coaching in the techniques of strength training. A well-trained staff will also provide guidance in using equipment and give helpful, supportive leadership during aerobics classes.

As you scout out clubs, look for those where the staff readily offers advice; you shouldn't have to ask for it. Also, be sure that all instructors are certified by one of the major fitness organizations (the American College of Sports Medicine, the American Council of Exercise, or the Aerobics and Fitness Association of America). You don't want Hanz and Franz experimenting on you.

PAIN IN THE POCKETBOOK

Don't let any gym give your wallet a workout. Remember, a long-term relationship with a good, affordable health club is better than a few months with a fancy club that busts your budget. Ask for a written list of membership options and a copy of the contract you would be signing. Never sign up on impulse! Take the information and contract home with you and review them carefully. If the salesperson tries to use high pressure such as "the deal is only good today," be wary. Ask if "the deal" can be extended a few days, or when it will be available again. Most clubs have running specials. Be the consummate tightwad and bargain over everything, especially initiation fees.

Avoid signing up for a multi-year membership; consider a month-to-month membership or one that lasts no longer than a year. This will give you the flexibility to change clubs if you decide that this one is not for you. It will also protect you in the event that the club goes out of business or changes ownership (it happens a lot). Most facilities have monthly payment plans that are easy on the pocketbook. Several national chains have reciprocal privileges with out-of-town/out-of-state facilities, so if you travel frequently you can train on the road at little or no additional cost.

INSPIRING AMBIENCE

It's a tried and true fact: If you don't feel comfortable in your gym, you're not going to make an effort to work out there. How you feel about a particular place can make all the difference in the world. Is the equipment well maintained and in working order? Is it clean and sanitary? Do you feel safe there? Is there adequate, well-lit parking? Does the staff make members feel welcome? Are you comfortable with the people you meet?

Choose a club as carefully as you would a mate. After all, you're going to be spending a lot of time there! If you want a light workout to pop music, you're not going to fit in at a hard-core bodybuilding gym. If you want an anonymous exercise experience, you

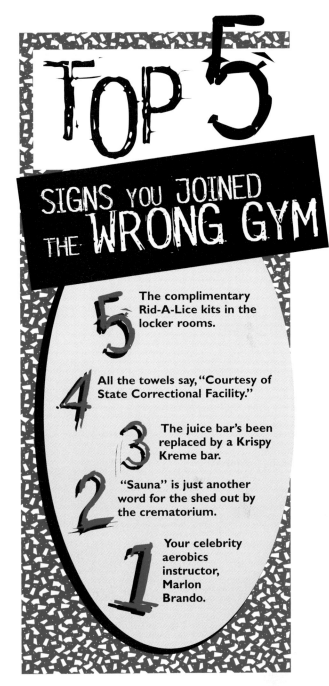

TOP 5 SIGNS YOU JOINED THE WRONG GYM

5 The complimentary Rid-A-Lice kits in the locker rooms.

4 All the towels say, "Courtesy of State Correctional Facility."

3 The juice bar's been replaced by a Krispy Kreme bar.

2 "Sauna" is just another word for the shed out by the crematorium.

1 Your celebrity aerobics instructor, Marlon Brando.

probably won't like the "see and be seen" atmosphere of a flashy chrome-and-neon club.

Joining a gym is a big commitment. It's a pledge of time, money, and effort. Health clubs have nothing to lose when your motivation wanes, so be true to yourself and choose wisely. The time you invest in shopping for the right health club will pay dividends in a pleasant workout that you will actually look forward to each day. And that's what it's all about!

EXERCISE ETIQUETTE,
OR: MISS (MUSCLE) MANNERS

Joining a health club can be confusing if you've never worked out much before. The miles and miles of machines, the hundreds of sweaty bodies pushing, pulling, and pumping—it can make you feel really like, uh, aroused, or inspired. Plus, you have to deal with all of those unwritten rules. What do you wear? How do you learn to work all those machines? What is the proper way to tell that man to stop napping on the leg press? Read on to learn the rules of exercise etiquette.

NAVIGATING YOUR GYM

Sure, it may look intimidating. All of those sweaty, lean bodies and their gleaming, bulging muscles. But if you can just get past the stack of *Fit* magazines in the reception area, you'll see that there's more to the gym than just mirrors and Spandex.

THE CARDIO AREA

See that machine with the moving belt? That's a treadmill, and it's for walking and/or running. And that one with the pedals? That's a stationary bike. See how easy this is? The first rule of thumb for using a cardio machine is the 20-Minute Law, to wit, don't stay on the machine for more than 20 minutes if there's a line. If

you break this rule, someone is going to kick you off and you will forever be marked as a "hogger." These people have already been waiting for 20 minutes, and they aren't happy, so watch out for dirty looks. For the record, once a hogger, always a hogger.

If you are waiting in line and the person you're eyeing has been trotting for 30 minutes, here's how to handle it. If you're comfortable with confrontation (and have a couple of muscle-bound friends backing you up), approach that person and say, "Pardon me, your running stride is great. But even perfection has to end, like about 10 minutes ago." If you don't feel comfortable with confrontation, find the club manager and ask her to take care of the clunkhead.

THE MACHINES

Now that you've conquered the cardio area (which doesn't just include treadmills by the way; there are dozens of cardio machines that work all kinds of muscles, including your heart), you must brave the Wide World of Resistance Machines. If you've never used machines before, they can be intimidating. Here's a little secret for you: Almost every machine in your gym has *instructions*. You might feel stupid reading the instructions, but won't you feel even more idiotic when everyone stares (and some people even applaud) when you somehow manage to do crunches on the leg extension machine?

Finally, wipe the sweat off the machine when you're done. It's just common courtesy. Not to mention, common frickin' sense.

THE FREE WEIGHTS

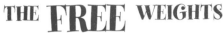

Gender is an issue in this part of the gym, so pay attention. Free weights are simply those that stand free as opposed to those that are part of a machine.

FOR WOMEN ONLY

The free weight section of the gym is a scary place. You'll see large groups of sweaty men grunting, groaning, and slinging sweat all over the place. Don't be afraid. They won't hurt you. If you don't know how to use the free weights, this is a great time to consider a personal trainer. If you know what you're doing, don't be afraid to saunter over there, grab your five-pound weights, and go to town. Women often feel intimidated by the presence of men in the free weight area but don't worry— they don't care what you're doing. They're too busy grunting and flexing to worry about little old you.

FOR MEN ONLY

Yes, you look manly and muscular with your 200-pound dumbbells, but take note: They're too heavy. The number one mistake most men make in the free weight department is lifting too much. Perhaps you're trying to impress everyone—no one can really explain this behavior. But throwing your weights down on the floor is a no-no and a big sign that your ego is bigger than your muscles. Here's a thought: Decrease the weight you lift or get a spotter. Everyone will marvel at your good sense.

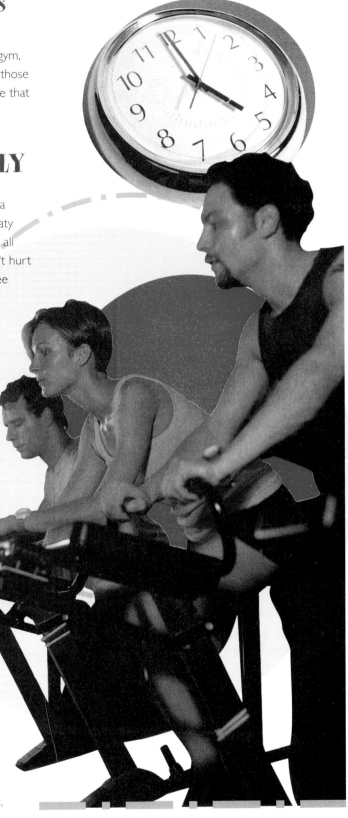

Deltoid DIARY

Getting in "Gear"

Okay, so I'm new to this whole fitness craze. I know, I know, it's been around forever so where have I been? I admit it. I have been hiding—rooted to the couch, glued to the TV, the comforter firmly in place over my head. I have stayed far away from anything that even resembles "healthy." Now, after successfully dodging the guilt, so to speak, I have been pulled, kicking and screaming, from my roost. I must exercise. I must eat right. I must pry my fat ass off the couch and face the music.

So, we will start at the beginning. I am *not* willing to give up my Cap'n Crunch, Devil Dogs, and cheese curls just yet. They tell me if I'm not willing to give up my favorite foods, all I have to do is work out enough to burn them off. Then I can eat as much as I want. That's a plan. How hard could it possibly be? Jump around a little bit, lift a few weights, no problem.

I head down to the gym on the corner, where I'm greeted at the door by an anorexically thin, depressingly cheerful girl a couple of years younger than I am. She leads me through the sign-up process and takes me on a tour of the "facilities." Locker rooms, weight rooms, aerobics class, swimming pool, steam rooms, saunas, and whirlpools. Our last stop is in front of a giant neon sign, shaped like a bicep; above it glow the words of

workout wisdom "Get in Gear!" Truly profound.

At this point, Bulimia Barbie says to me, "Like, do you have any gear?" I look puzzled. "You know, like workout clothes, like what I'm wearing."

You call tights and dental floss "clothes?" And when did clothing become "gear"? I cautiously step inside the gym store and am immediately inundated by images of sickeningly slim females and bulging biceps hanging on every inch of spare wall space. A pounding, booming beat, like some collective giant heart, seems to control every move. Once again, I am greeted by an incredibly thin girl, dressed in what looks like a bra and panties. (Are they cloning these chicks?)

"Hi! Are you looking for some gear?" I tell her I'm just gear browsing and move to the opposite side of the store.

As I peruse the selection, I see more of what I've seen on the clones working here, just in different colors. Why do they make these things so tiny? Wouldn't it make sense that if you need "gear" in the first place, then you also need to work out? If you need to work out, you probably don't have the best shape. If you don't have the best shape, you certainly don't want to try to squeeze it into one of those tiny little suits.

I finally find something that I might consider wearing in public and head for the dressing room. I strip and try to squash myself into this Spandex Lycra leotard thing. I have it pulled so tight and stretched so far, I hope I don't lose my grip; it might snap back and launch me into space! Okay, I think I've got the straps over my shoulders, but wait. What's that hanging out the bottom? All right, tuck that in. Oops, it popped out the top. Shove that back in. By this time the clone is outside the door: "How are we doing?"

I turn and look at myself in the full-length mirror (this is why I don't own one of these things!), wiggle out of this horrible torture device, and open the door. I drop the misshapen piece of Lycra into the clone's hands and walk past her.

"Cash or charge?"

Yeah, right! I'm going home.

That was enough of a workout for me. I'm going back to my safe couch and my beautiful, relaxing TV, and there I'll exercise—my option, that is, to watch another rousing episode on the *E!* channel.

25 EASY WAYS TO GET YOUR EXERCISE

- 25 Beating around the bush
- 24 Climbing the walls
- 23 Swallowing your pride
- 22 Passing the buck
- 21 Throwing your weight around
- 20 Dragging your heels
- 19 Going over the edge
- 18 Picking up the pieces
- 17 Making mountains out of molehills
- 16 Wading through paperwork
- 15 Bending over backwards
- 14 Jumping on the bandwagon
- 13 Balancing the books
- 12 Running around in circles
- 11 Pushing your luck
- 10 Eating crow
- 9 Tooting your own horn
- 8 Climbing the ladder of success
- 7 Pulling out all the stops
- 6 Adding fuel to the fire
- 5 Opening a can of worms
- 4 Putting your foot in your mouth
- 3 Hitting the nail on the head
- 2 Starting the ball rolling
- 1 Jumping through hoops

Deltoid DIARY

Sauna Shave

As the ball made its final victorious thud against the wall, I could sense my opponent conceding to my athletic prowess. Hungry for another win, I could feel all eyes on me as I sidled over to my adversary for the obligatory handshake. Racquetball was my game, my calling card, and nothing stood in my way as I chalked up another win for (insert Queen's "We Are the Champions" here) ME.

Riding high on my latest accomplishment, I sauntered over to the water fountain, downed a couple of gulps of refreshing water, and made a stop at the showers.

As the water worked its magic on my weary muscles, I mentally rehashed some of my ingenious maneuvers on the court and smiled as I recalled the look of doom from my rival. Victory was mine, yet again, and today was my day to shine. After the shower, it was time to claim my own personal reward: a refreshing, relaxing moment in the sauna.

This was a perk that I saved for such special occasions, a time when nothing could or would disturb me as I attempted to escape reality, if only for 10 minutes. Making that final stroll was a momentous occasion, and I welcomed the quiet that would greet me as I sat in the dry heat and became enveloped in its comfort.

But there was a slight problem. A naked, obese, hairy mess holding a disposable razor stood in the way. There he sat, alone, in all his naked, immensely unfit splendor, dutifully shaving to and fro. And as he continued to slather on the shaving cream in some pretty disgusting nooks and crannies, I could feel my dream of steamy bliss drifting away from me.

There is more. The lifeless hairs were suddenly sprawled all around the sauna benches, floors, and drain, and there seemed to be no end to them. I watched this mess from the sauna door window, with one hand on the door handle, the other stranded somewhere in mid-air, with my facial features stuck in a permanent scowl. This unclothed beast (truly a Fat Bastard) stood between me and well deserved quietude.

As my senses returned to me and I released the grip I had on the sauna door handle, it became clear that this transgressor was not going to leave. The thought of witnessing his act again made me nauseous. Welcome to the public gym, I thought, and all its (hairless) humanity.

PECTORALIS MAJOR, OR: CONFESSIONS OF A PERSONAL TRAINER

Just around the corner from the juice bar and between the water fountain and the rest rooms is a tiny broom-sized office reserved for that favored of all fitness experts, the personal trainer. Not everyone can afford a personal trainer, but that's not what's stopping most people from visiting these pectoralis majors. The fact is, most of us would prefer to get our fitness advice from an article in a magazine or a *1-Minute Abs* video rather than from a real, live, physically fit human being who will no doubt take one look at our cottage cheese thighs and beer bellies, smirk, and say, "So, eat much?"

But take heart, not all of these personal trainers have a chip on their bulging, twitching shoulder muscles. We've found one who's willing to come clean about what's right, and what's wrong, with her clientele:

I can tell by the first sentence that comes out of your mouth whether you'll succeed or not. Your body language, your history, your past, and your attitude—they all speak volumes about you. The way you stand, the way you sit, the way you hold a dumbbell, and even the way you walk from the front door to the personal training office tells me what I need to know before you even say a thing.

No, I don't have ESP. What I do have is experience, and that counts for a lot in this business. In an hour I have to determine your fitness level, biomechanical weaknesses, medical and fitness history, body fat, workout preferences, and, most important, your reasons for meeting with me in the first place.

Are you sitting here because you joined the gym and then realized that there are about 400 machines you'll never figure out on your own? Or do you have an injury you're recovering from and you don't know how to rehab it? Maybe you want to lose 30 pounds before your wedding next spring, or maybe you're simply tired of doing the same old workout and need something new. Whatever it is, your reason for sitting here is more important than anything else I could find out about you. Here I've detailed, from worst to best, the attitudes that will make or break your commitment to get in shape.

WORST ATTITUDE

"I've Tried Everything, but I Just Can't Seem to Lose Any Weight!"

ATTITUDE ADJUSTMENT NEEDED:
Complete Mental Overhaul

I don't know how many times I've heard someone say this. When someone sits down and launches into detail about the diets they've tried and the books they've read and the contraptions they've bought, I know I'm in trouble. Oh, I don't doubt their sincerity—I *know* they're desperate to lose weight. But it's that desperation that's going to make nine out of ten of these people quit before they've even really started.

If you've said this before, either to your best friend, your trainer, or your dog, you've got some serious work to do.

Why? When you say this, you generally want to lose weight, and you want to lose it right now. You'll nod solemnly when I explain that safe, permanent weight loss happens only with exercise and a healthy diet—not just for a few weeks, but forever. In the next breath you'll tell me that you *never* eat breakfast for fear of getting fat. You'll eagerly agree to my workout schedule and then, at your next appointment, you'll spend 10 minutes explaining why you couldn't get to the gym at all that week. If you don't have a serious change of attitude, chances are I won't be seeing you around the gym after our sessions are over, and you probably won't return any of my calls.

THE SOLUTION

You know what your problem is? You're relying on your willpower to deliver the goods. As has been stated in numerous fitness books, trusting in willpower to alter bad health habits is like believing the tooth fairy really delivers dollar bills.

Willpower only lasts for about a day or two, if you're lucky, and when it slinks away, you're going straight back to Burger King, kicking yourself all the way. It's the long run you need to be thinking about, which means, first of all, making the commitment to be healthier. Once you've made that commitment, figure out what you're doing wrong. If you don't know what you're doing wrong, how can you change it?

Then set some small goals. You say you want to lose body fat? Instead of reducing your daily calorie intake to 100 calories of rice cakes, how about simply cutting out that donut you eat every morning? That alone will save you at least 300 calories and lots of fat grams too. When you've conquered the Bad Donut Habit, move on to conquer the next bad habit. You need a real lifestyle change.

harsh realities to let go of my dream to be cellulite- and pooch-free, and so will you.

Luckily, you're not a lost cause. You're simply under the delusion that you can get rid of that pooch and that cellulite. I'm not saying it's impossible, but chances are, if you're this close to your "ideal weight," you're already working out on a regular basis and aware of the right foods to eat. You're a healthy eater and you probably spend four or five days in the gym doing aerobics and lifting weights. You're strong, you have relatively low body fat, and you look pretty damn good in a bathing suit. So why are you here? I can hear you right now saying, "You know, if you could just show me some better ab exercise, I'm *sure* I'll finally get that six pack." Don't worry, we'll get ya fixed up.

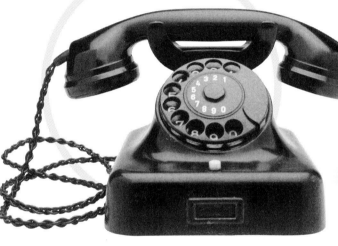

SLIGHTLY **BAD** ATTITUDE

"I Just Need to Lose Ten More Pounds."

ATTITUDE ADJUSTMENT NEEDED:
Slight

Have you ever said this? Don't be shy, we've all thought this at one time or another. I've heard so many healthy and beautiful women say that very thing to me it's bewildering. If you've ever uttered those words, you're probably worried about that lower-belly pooch that just won't go away, or the cellulite that clings to your rear with the tenacity of an outer space alien. I know all about those worries, because I have them too.

The only difference is, I had to deal with some

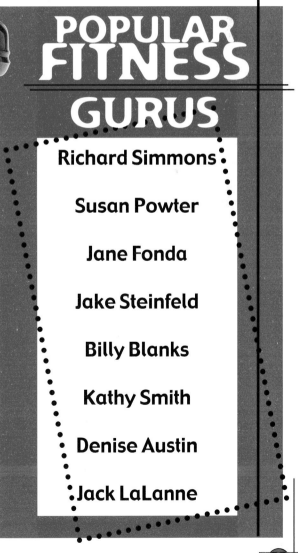

POPULAR FITNESS GURUS

Richard Simmons

Susan Powter

Jane Fonda

Jake Steinfeld

Billy Blanks

Kathy Smith

Denise Austin

Jack LaLanne

THE SOLUTION

There's nothing wrong with wanting to lose a few more pounds and, as your trainer, I'm going to look at your current workouts and eating habits and we're going to come up with a plan. First of all, you should vary your cardio workouts so that you have some medium-intensity workouts and some high-intensity workouts. Change the kind of exercise you're doing, the length, the intensity, and the frequency and you'll start burning more calories.

Keep in mind, you may not even lose much more weight. Your body has a settling point and, when you reach it, it doesn't want to budge. So, you'll either accept your beautifully strong body, flaws and all, or you'll call up the local plastic surgeon for a look-see. Either way, you'll be set with a little bit of work or a few cuts, okay?

BEST ATTITUDE

"I Don't Care How Much Weight I Lose. I Just Want More Energy."

ATTITUDE ADJUSTMENT NEEDED:
—*None*

Whoever you are, I love you when you say this to me. If you walk into my office, hold your head high, laugh when you see the body fat measurement, and then shrug when I detail the workout I have planned for you, you're the winner. You're probably already exercising, maybe a light walk every day or a swim. You might not have any experience with weights, but you're pretty much game for anything. You eat moderate portions of what you like and don't worry about the occasional candy bar or hamburger. You're secure in yourself and you'll probably work with me regularly for the next year or so.

Then we're both winners.

EASY exercises:

Step UP!

Using a step or something similar, step up alternating your leading leg every 30 seconds (i.e., 30 seconds leading with the right leg and then 30 seconds leading with the left). Keep your back straight and make sure your whole foot is on top of the step each time you step up. When you step down again, keep close to the step and use your arms.

Muscle Myth:
Exercising takes too much time.

Triceps Truth:
Regular exercise doesn't have to take much more than 15 to 30 minutes, three or four times a week.

Squats

Begin by standing up straight with your feet shoulder-width apart and toes facing forward. Bend your knees and push your bottom away from you as you squat down, keeping your heels pressed to the floor. To help perform the squat correctly, pretend you're going to sit down into an imaginary chair. If you wish, you can also hold a weighted bar across your shoulders to make the squat even harder. Straighten your knees again and stand upright to return to the starting position.

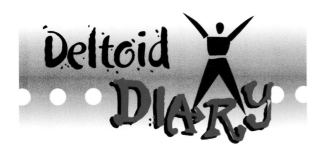

Working Workout

Working at a gym has its benefits. Free membership with no restrictions. Convenient access to the latest health and fitness information. A friendly working atmosphere. Oh, and a passport to all the juicy, shocking, and disturbing gossip you can handle.

Yep. Working at a health club also includes being counselor, dietitian, social worker, confidante, personal consultant—the list goes on and on. But one of the hats to be worn bestows a special honor on the health club receptionist. This role means hearing about the unusual acts of fellow gym goers, and in order to appease the membership, finding a solution.

For example, one such story involves a little old lady partaking in a high impact aerobics class without underwear. That's as in: absolutely no underwear. We are talking some very old breasts gleefully swaying around without any support; and while the unaware senior citizen sits on the ground, obediently following the leader's strides, she puts on display her, ahem, lower half for her neighbor's viewing pleasure. Paints quite an attractive picture,

doesn't it? Try maintaining composure while clients rehash every move this unshackled grandma makes in the latest Tae Bo class.

Then there are the endless stories involving acts of nudity. Like when a person is greeted by a naked lady reading a magazine in the sauna with her legs propped up. Try telling such a person that they should act more appropriately. Then there are the cries of overpriced dues and unsatisfactory amenities that send you running for the safety of your work cubicle.

Of course, no health club receptionist's day is complete without hearing about an undetectable odor originating from the locker room. It is enough to make you wonder if a competing gym is plotting against you. But the reality is that people tend to view their local gym as a place where they suspend their normal behavior. What else can explain how seemingly

decent, clean people can spend an evening at the gym showing less control than a five-year-old? Toilet paper somehow finds its way strewn throughout the place, stale food is stashed in lockers, and newly posted informational signs are shredded to bits, all in a matter of hours.

The gym receptionist is not merely a greeter, or a poster child for ideal health; no, her duties go way beyond that. You learn far more about members than you ever wanted to know. So the next time you are at the gym, and you witness the receptionist fielding requests for different music or installing more toilet paper, make sure you stop and thank him or her for a job well done. And ask about the latest gossip!

DRESS CODE DILEMMA, OR: SPANDEX SECRETS

The whole idea of wearing proper gym attire is important, so please read these instructions carefully.

LADIES (DAY AND) NIGHT

Skimpy clothing is pretty much a staple of most health clubs, and that's not a bad thing. If you've worked hard at your routine and have a great butt to show for it, by all means, show it off. Wear Spandex or tights, if you must, and be proud of it. But, for the record, thongs, leotards, and legwarmers are *out*. Even men don't want to see you wearing them, so if you're still

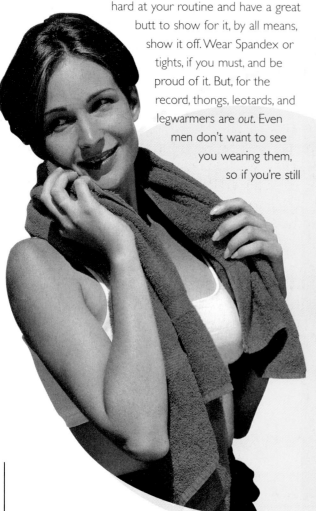

using Jane Fonda's first video as a guide to workout attire, you should probably update your video collection. (Not to mention your wardrobe.)

In the same vein, makeup is a no-no. If you're coming straight from work, it's understandable for you to have the work version of hair and makeup. But, if it's 5:00 a.m., there's no reason for you to be dolled up and, as soon as you start sweating, it's going to go all over the place anyway. This only serves to make *you* look out of place. Unless you work out at the local clown school, that is.

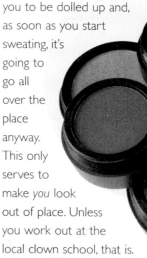

Lest you think you *have* to wear something skin-tight just to work out, please note that it's also perfectly acceptable to dress in your best skank-clothes. The gym is the only place in the world (other than homeless shelters) that allows mismatching neon outfits in tandem with holey shirts and stained shorts. Where else but on the treadmill will you feel perfectly at ease in your painting-the-house clothes?

When you're a new exerciser, you tend to worry about things like matching your sports bra to your socks. This is perfectly normal and will soon pass. In the meantime, you'll find yourself at the store agonizing over which outfit is the coolest. As you get the hang of this exercise stuff, you'll find that comfort is king in the gym. You'll want to wear things that cover all your delicate parts and won't fly open when you wedge yourself into the leg press or send your legs skyward for some crunches. You want clothes that don't ride, pinch, or squeeze and, most important, you want quality clothes than can withstand daily washings.

One other important point: Do *not*, under any circumstances, wear pantyhose underneath your shorts. If you need an explanation for this rule, seek counseling.

WHAT TO WEAR TO THE GYM

OK

T-shirts
comfortable shorts
sports bra
gloves
tube socks
gym shoes

WHAT NOT TO WEAR TO THE GYM

clown makeup
plastic muscles
giant afro wig
clothing of the opposite gender
shoes that are two sizes too big
shorts that are two sizes too small
Spandex shorts
nothing

GENTLEMAN'S (HEALTH) CLUB

One word: package. No one wants to see it. Spandex on men at the gym is the equivalent of wearing a Speedo on the beach; it's disgusting and all the women are going to make fun of you for wearing it. Once you know you are the butt, so to speak, of other's ridicule, the rest of the fashion guessing game will be a piece of cake.

Men are simple creatures and, as such, don't have to worry about silly things like matching outfits and questionable taste. In fact, there are almost no rules for men's fashion in a health club except the

Spandex horror just mentioned, and sweatpants. In general, the gym is just about the only acceptable place to wear sweatpants, aside from behind closed doors where only your girlfriend will be offended (and she will, make no mistake). This doesn't mean that warm-ups are a no-no; a nice pair of *baggy* striped sweatpants will get you lots of close female scrutiny. However, sweatpants that reveal every crease, crevice, and bulge of your body will put you on the oh-god-don't-look-at-that-guy-over-there list currently circulating among female gym goers everywhere.

Your best bet is to get several pairs of baggy shorts and lots of stinky T-shirts. Oh, you already have those? Then you're all set.

PECTORALIS PACKING,
OR: LUNGE LUGGAGE

The gym bag comes in as many shapes and sizes as gym goers. However, what is in the perfect gym bag? The answer to that depends on the needs of the owner. Do you run in, work out, and go home, or do you need to head to the office afterward?

CARDIO QUESTIONS

Several variables determine what you should pack in your bag. They are:

• What do you need to work out?
• Are you going to shower at the gym?
• Do you need to clean up and go to work afterward?
• Do you have a locker where you can store items on a long-term basis?

LIMBER UP LIST

Before you pack your gym bag, you need to figure out what items you need to have with you in order to have a successful workout. Regardless of how long or short, easy or strenuous a workout is, be sure to carry a small towel to wipe down the equipment after using it. Do not be surprised if you end up using it to wipe the previous person's slime off the equipment before you use it as well. Nobody wants to slip and slide in another's discharge. In most gyms, a towel is required. Some gyms will not even permit you past the check-in desk without proving you have one with you. Some will even require you to purchase or rent one from the facility; better clubs have them available throughout the gym.

BODY BASICS

Start with the basics. Will you wear your workout clothes and shoes to the gym, or will you need to bring them with you? Even if you wear your workout clothes, you may choose to pack your shoes so you do not get them covered with mud or worse when walking outside the gym. If you wear your exercise clothes, you will probably need to change into street clothes when you are finished. If you need to pack your street clothes, be sure to roll them tightly. This will keep them from wrinkling, and they will take up less room as well. Be sure to remember everything you'll need. For instance, it is really awful to forget clean underwear if you have to go to work later, and then have to take a client to lunch. ("Uh, I think that smell is the broccoli, sir.")

Another basic, yet important item is your water bottle. It is extremely important to stay hydrated while working out. This is especially true if you are taking muscle-enhancing sup- plements that dehydrate you or eating meal supple- ment bars that need to be taken with plenty of water.

Remember, it takes time to walk over to the water fountain, which probably is not dispensing mountain spring water anyway.

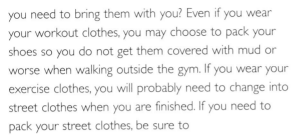

Make sure you mark your bottle with your name to avoid accidentally picking up and drinking someone else's water. (Or worse, one of those god-awful protein shakes!)

PERSONAL (STUFF) MATTERS

Do not forget to pack your personal exercise equipment. If you use gloves, a back support, a tutu, or any other stuff, these should have a permanent place in your gym bag. However, this does not mean they do not need to be taken out periodically and cleaned as needed (hint, hint). A rule of thumb: If after removing your hands from your gloves they smell worse than the inside of your shoes, you may want to consider getting a new pair. However, as long as your equipment is not offensive smelling and is in good repair, you are okay.

WHAT TO PACK IN A GYM BAG

towel
weight lifting gloves
bottle of water
Power Bar
change of clothes
portable CD player
vitamins/supplements
weightlifting belt
ankle/wrist weights
Gatorade

MUSIC (REALLY) MATTERS!

Do you like to rock out to music while you work out? Do people stop just to see what is referred to (behind your back) as the spastic dance? So pack your anti-shock CD player. You should also pack several CDs. Keep them in some sort of container to protect them from moisture and damage. Pack an extra set of batteries as well. The only thing worse than not having any music to get spastic with is having no juice to crank your player.

LOCKER LESSONS

Regardless of whether you have an assigned long-term locker or if you pick a different temporary locker every time you go to the health club, you will need a lock. Invest in a good one. Always use a combination-type

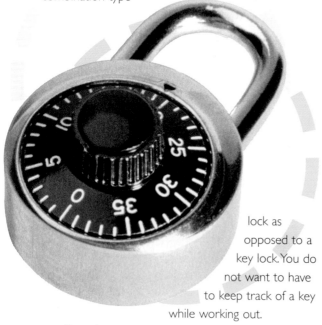

lock as opposed to a key lock. You do not want to have to keep track of a key while working out.

If you have trouble remembering your combination, here's a hint: Do not write it on your hand. Sweat is an excellent ink remover. Write it on a piece of masking tape and stick it in your shoe. Remove it once you have committed it to memory. Which will never happen.

EASY exercises:

Lower-Leg Lift

Lie on your side with your head resting in your hand and the top leg resting on the ground in front of you. To work your inner thigh area, raise your lower leg off the floor toward a 45-degree angle. Make sure you don't lift your leg too high. When you lower your leg, keep it just above the floor and avoid resting it between lifts. Roll over and work the inner thigh of the other leg for the same amount of time.

Plate Crunch

Lie on your back on the floor with your knees slightly bent and your heels on the floor. Place a light weight plate or dumbbell on your chest and hold it by crossing your arms over it. Contract your abdominals and lift your torso. Use the abdominals to lift the weight on your upper body. Curl up and down slowly, concentrating on the contraction of the abdominal muscles.

TOTALLY TOILETRIES

Once you have finished working out, what do you do? Do you use the shower, sauna, or hot tub? Do you leave in your workout clothes and go home, or do you change into your street clothes and go to work? Whatever you do, if you take off your shoes and socks and walk around for any reason, you need shower slippers or flip-flops. If you do not wear some sort of protective footwear, you will be walking on varieties of foot fungus that can dissolve a toenail. You should wear shoes everywhere in the locker room, the shower, the toilet stalls, the sauna, and to and from the hot tub. The floor of the locker room, even if cleaned daily, is teeming with mad scientist germs.

IF THE (BATHING) SUIT FITS

If you plan to use the gym's pool, hot tub, or sauna, pack a bathing suit. Some people are comfortable going nude into the sauna and hot tub. Then again, some people don't know what they look like naked. The basic rule: Cover it or them or whatever you have.

TOWEL TROUBLES

Some gyms provide towels for the locker room, sauna, hot tub, and/or pool at no cost or at a nominal fee. Most, however, do not provide towels. Even if your gym does provide them, it is a good idea to bring your own. You may need one to sit on for the drive home if you do not have enough time to shower. It is much easier to wash a towel than have your car seat steam cleaned.

If you will be getting ready for work or to go out after the gym, you will need to pack everything you need to clean up. Some gyms have vending machines for toiletries. It helps to place all of your toiletries in a separate plastic bag or container in case of leaks.

BATHING BASICS

Some gyms have soap dispensers in the showers. However, if they are empty or you have sensitive skin, you will need to provide your own. Liquid soap will store in your bag or locker much easier than bar soap. If you have to carry it around with you, remember to secure the pump before placing it in your bag. You do not want to soil everything else in your gym bag. Everything else you should be able to figure out.

(SPARE) CHANGE WILL DO YOU GOOD

Some miscellaneous items you may want to carry include $2 in change for a vending machine. If you forget your water bottle, you can usually buy a bottle of water or sports drink for $2 or less. Do not put anything of great value in your bag or locker. Do not keep your valuable jewelry or large amounts of cash in your bag or locker while you work out. If possible, place them in the management's safe-deposit box or leave them at home.

POPULAR EXERCISE ACCESSORIES

- weight lifting belt
- sports bra
- jock strap
- sweat socks
- weight lifting gloves
- stopwatch
- sweatband
- gym bag

TAE-BO TO GO

While training in his home one fateful day, martial arts expert, boxing pro, action movie star, and all-around he-man Billy Blanks decided to combine energetic dance music with his regular round of challenging Tae Kwon Do moves. This decision, and the resulting action-packed fitness routine, eventually evolved into the cultural and physical phenomenon known simply as Tae-Bo. Billy soon saw what Tae-Bo did for himself and his own family, so in 1989 he opened the Billy Blanks World Training Center in California. Eventually, sometime during the mid '90s, the rest of the world caught on and Billy was coaxed into making the first Tae-Bo video, which would change the way the world thought about exercise videos.

Perhaps Billy's movie roles as a tough-talking but even harder kicking martial arts expert and all-around tough guy in such Hollywood hits as *The Last Boy Scout* and *Kiss the Girls*, not to mention in hard-core, hard-hitting action flicks like *Lion Heart* and *Expect No Mercy*, were a training ground of sorts for his eventual rise to exercise video superstardom as the Jane Fonda of the '90s. Either way, no one can deny the cultural, not to mention physical, benefits of the Tae-Bo training system. Four videos strong and still growing like America's newly sleek leg muscles, Tae-Bo is here to stay.

BUT What THE HECK IS TAE-BO?

Tae-Bo is a unique and challenging fitness workout resulting from a martial arts/aerobics hybrid created by Billy Blanks as far back as the late '70s. (Talk about patience being a virtue!) When performed properly (as in not wimping out and stopping the tape halfway through), Tae-Bo combines the challenging trio of Tae Kwon Do, boxing, and dance disciplines and puts them together in an exhausting program choreographed to the refreshing and energetic strains of thumping hip-hop music. A typical one-hour routine (come on, you can make it) consists of a series of jabs, punches, kicks, and dance steps, set to music in a series of eight-count combinations.

The name, Tae-Bo, is a combination of other words: "Tae" means "leg" and it relates to the kicks and lower body part of the workout. "Bo" comes from boxing and the upper body punches that are an integral part of the workout. Part of the popularity of Tae-Bo is that it can be a very satisfying, all-in-one work-out because it engages the entire body instead of focusing on just one muscle group such as other videos like *8 Minute Abs* and *Buns of Steel*.

YEAH, BUT IS TAE-BO FOR ME?

Sure it is. In fact, the vast appeal of Tae-Bo is that it is for anyone who wants a complete and satisfying workout. From the tips of your totally tapping toes to the top of your ducking and weaving head, Tae-Bo offers a walloping workout for the entire body.

The best part? Tae-Bo can be done at your own pace. With its rapidly evolving series of videos, from the first Tae-Bo to Tae-Bo Gold, you can achieve physical nirvana right in your very own home. (This includes the popular "pause while you go to the bathroom or chug a bottle of water" option, formerly unavailable in most fitness clubs.) As you build strength, you can do more and you can increase your level of physical fitness.

On the other hand, just like the generic terms jazzercise and aerobics, the concepts of Tae-Bo are now taught by Billy Blanks stand-ins all across the country. Trade in your videos, not to mention your living room, for a live, interactive workout with trained instructors and a class full of everyone from experts to beginners.

HOW FAST DOES IT WORK?

As with any other exercise program or fitness routine, results vary. Naturally, if you've never worked out, let alone done Tae-Bo, before, you'll definitely feel "something" after your very first session. Whether you feel it in the emergency room or the locker room afterward is up to you and your level of common sense. However, don't go into Tae-Bo, or any other fitness program for that matter, expecting immediate results. Hard work and dedication are as much a part of the Tae-Bo philosophy as comfortable shoes and a VCR. Just buying the tape or signing up for the class isn't enough. Allow yourself to be swept up by the Tae-Bo philosophy, the thumping bass, and Billy Blanks's

infectious yet paternal coaching, and you should start to see results after several weeks.

DO I HAVE TO DO TAE-BO EVERY DAY?

Again, common sense, and books such as this, tell you to check with your physician before you start any intense workout program. According to your personal level of fitness, the amount of rest you give your body, and the level of intensity you put into each and every workout, Tae-Bo can be done every day or as little as a couple of times a week. For maximum benefit, like any other cardiovascular program of course, you should consider doing Tae-Bo at least three times a week for minimum results.

Naturally, beginners to both exercise in general and Tae-Bo in particular are advised to start slow and build up their endurance. Tae-Bo is a challenging yet rewarding workout and as such requires the use of your entire body. Don't get discouraged if you get tired quickly in the beginning. The whole idea of Tae-Bo is to maximize the benefits by incorporating the entire body into the workout.

DOES TAE-BO REQUIRE ANY SPECIAL EQUIPMENT?

Aside from a VCR and one, or all, of the Tae-Bo videotapes, the answer to this question is "not really." As with most workouts, comfortable clothing and appropriate footwear are also recommended, although extras like boxing gloves, those catchy red and yellow Tae-Bo headbands, and a stopwatch to check your heart rate are optional.

Of course, your second option is to join a gym and sign up for one or all of the almost daily Tae-Bo classes, which will require a gym membership, plenty of time, and a qualified instructor, not to mention the above comfortable clothes and appropriate footwear.

5

EXERCISING
YOUR RIGHTS (AND LEFTS)

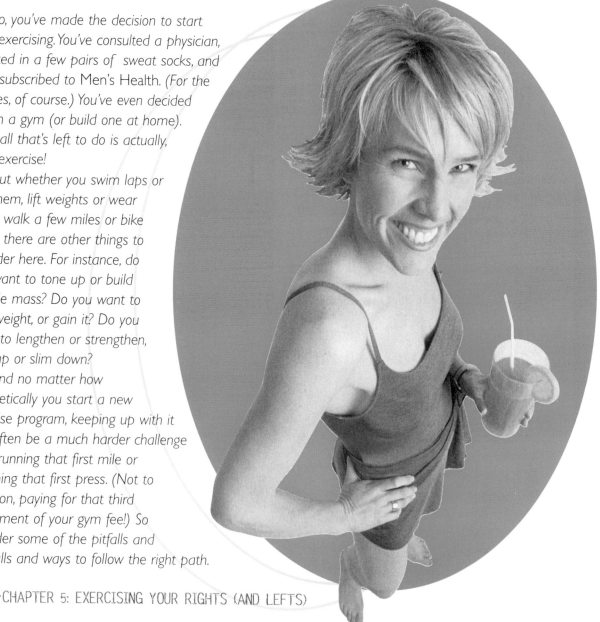

So, you've made the decision to start exercising. You've consulted a physician, invested in a few pairs of sweat socks, and even subscribed to Men's Health. (For the articles, of course.) You've even decided to join a gym (or build one at home). Now all that's left to do is actually, gulp, exercise!

But whether you swim laps or run them, lift weights or wear them, walk a few miles or bike them, there are other things to consider here. For instance, do you want to tone up or build muscle mass? Do you want to lose weight, or gain it? Do you want to lengthen or strengthen, firm up or slim down?

And no matter how energetically you start a new exercise program, keeping up with it can often be a much harder challenge than running that first mile or benching that first press. (Not to mention, paying for that third installment of your gym fee!) So consider some of the pitfalls and pratfalls and ways to follow the right path.

BABY (FAT) STEPS, OR: KNOWLEDGE IS POWER (BARS)

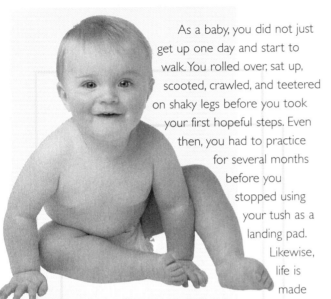

As a baby, you did not just get up one day and start to walk. You rolled over, sat up, scooted, crawled, and teetered on shaky legs before you took your first hopeful steps. Even then, you had to practice for several months before you stopped using your tush as a landing pad. Likewise, life is made up of baby steps. When beginning a new fitness program, you need to start slowly. This is a lifestyle change. You need to learn how to exercise, how to eat properly, and how to break bad habits. If you expect perfection, you can also expect to fail. The keys to success are motivation, knowledge, patience, dedication, discipline, and flexibility. Before you get started, you should realize one thing: There are no get-fit-quick schemes that work. Shaping your body, nonsurgically, takes time and hard work. Give yourself about two to four weeks to see results. If you plan carefully, getting fit can be fun and rewarding.

This is your program, so make it fun.

FIT PHYSICIAN

The first thing you should do before beginning any fitness program is consult your doctor. You have probably seen this advice before. It is probably the most ignored advice ever given. However, it is very important to consult your physician, especially if you have or have had health or physical issues, you have not exercised for a long period, you have not had a physical within the past 12 months, or you are severely overweight.

Your doctor can recommend any needed exercise modifications or conditions for your current health status.

For instance, if you have a bad back or a trick knee, deadlifting large amounts of weight is probably not the best exercise for you. Further, if you have low blood sugar, it may be necessary for you to eat a special diet. Your doctor can also recommend any needed dietary supplements or vitamins.

GREAT WORKOUT SONGS

"Flashdance (What a Feeling)," Irene Cara

"Maniac," Michael Sembello

"Physical," Olivia Newton-John

"Baby Workout," Jackie Wilson

"Workbench Workout," Sonic Boom

"Jump Around," House of Pain

"Shake, Rattle & Roll," Jerry Lee Lewis

"Fat," Weird Al Yankovic

MUSCLE MAP

Once you have a clean bill of health, or at least a workable arrangement, you are ready to map out your fitness plan. Decide what your goals are and what your timeline is. For instance, do you want to lose 20 pounds within 3 months? Despite those diet center commercials, you will probably not lose 100 pounds in 6 months. It is neither healthy or advisable to lose weight too rapidly. It is very strenuous on your heart. Two pounds per week is a healthy and realistic goal.

Be very specific with your goals. This will help you stay focused on what you need to do. Break down your ultimate goal into smaller goals. Every time you reach a smaller goal, you will feel motivated to keep going.

TRICEPS TIME

Another important factor in mapping out your program is time. How much time per day or per week do you have to dedicate to exercising? If you want to lose weight, you will need to do at least 30 minutes of aerobic exercise where your heart rate is in the target zone at least 3 times per week. Consult your physician or gym trainer to determine what your target zone heart rate is. Depending on what your goals are and what form of exercise you are doing, you may also need to incorporate time to do strength muscle workouts. For example, if you are going to walk or jog and you also want a toned upper body, you will also need to schedule time to work your upper body. You may walk or jog 3 times per week for 30 minutes and lift weights 3 times per week. Unless you are planning to spend several hours every day working out, most exercise needs can be broken down and worked into almost every schedule. You just need to be creative.

You can walk for 30 minutes at lunch, and then lift weights or do strength exercises at home or in the gym after work. You can also walk or jog one day, and then do your strength exercises the next day. It all depends on you and your needs. As long as you do your aerobics in blocks of at least 30 minutes and give your muscles adequate time to rest between strength training or weightlifting, you will be fine.

EASY exercise: MARCH in PLACE

March in place while sitting or standing up, bringing your knees as high as possible for the most health benefits. Work up to 5 minutes for this exercise to really be effective. This exercises both your hips and your knees.

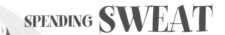

SPENDING SWEAT

Once you figure out how much time you have to exercise, you need to decide how you want to spend it. Find something that interests you. If you get bored or dislike your exercise, you will not do it for very long. There are many avenues to explore, so do not feel locked in to your choice. There are three main exercise mediums: gym, home, and sports. Do not feel like you must go to a gym in order to have an exercise program. If a gym is not for you, you can work out at home or play a sport. There are more exercise videos than you can shake a chicken leg at—everything from Tai Chi to funk aerobics to kickboxing. There is something for everyone and for every level.

You can also rent most titles from a video store before investing in them. Further, you can create a small home gym with little money and little space. All you need to start with is a small set of dumbbells, some ankle weights, and maybe a jump rope.

However, if you are interested in a sport, then that might be where your fitness interest lies. You do not have to think only of traditional sports like running, football, or baseball. You can also bike ride, inline skate, or power walk, not to mention indoor rock climbing or surfing. If it interests you, look into it.

EASY exercise: Sitting Stomach Crunches

Sitting erect, press the small of your back against the back of a chair while tightening your stomach muscles. Repeat several times. This exercises your back and stomach muscles.

SAVING PACE

Regardless of how you choose to exercise, you must start out slowly and at the proper level. If you have never put on a pair of Roller Blades, a bad place to start is at the top of the biggest hill in your city. If you have never lifted weights before, do not expect yourself to deadlift 300 pounds. Also, avoid worrying about keeping up in an aerobics class. It is better to do the exercise correctly one time than to do it incorrectly ten times. If you have not exercised in a while, give yourself time to get adjusted. Do the easiest course, lift the smallest weights, or use the beginner's videotape. If you try to do something you are not ready for, you risk getting discouraged and even injured.

The trick is to start slowly and master your exercise one step at a time. You want your program to be fun and effective. Flailing is not making the most of your exercise time or energy. It is also embarrassing. Arnold Schwarzenegger did not start off lifting 300-pound weights. He started slowly. If you see someone who is obviously skilled at the exercise or sport you have chosen, do not be afraid to ask him/her for pointers. The only way you will learn is by asking questions and experimenting. Do not be afraid to fall down or fail. You only really fail if you quit.

A good way to keep track of your program and your goals is to use a calendar. In pencil, write down each of your goals on the corresponding dates. Again, be realistic about your goals. In addition to writing down your goals, schedule your workout times. Make it clear to yourself that your program is important enough to write down. Do not just write "Exercise." Write down exactly what you plan to do on each day, and then go back and write down exactly what you did. This will help you keep track of how well you are keeping to your fitness plan as well as how well your fitness plan is working. If you are missing workouts or not completing what you thought you should, evaluate your program and make any needed changes. You have written your entries in pencil for a reason. Your program should not feel like a prison. Be flexible enough to change what is not working, but dedicated enough to work through the tough times.

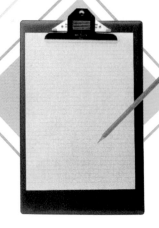

"Start slow and taper off."
—Walt Stack, marathon runner

SETBACK SHUFFLE

When you experience a setback, and you will, it is not the end of the world. Setbacks are an important part of the process. They are very telling. For instance, you can see if it is your program that needs to be changed, or your attitude. If you are missing workout appointments because you run out of time or energy during the day, you need to change when you schedule them. However, if you are missing them because you do not feel like doing them, you need to think about why you started in the first place, regroup, and start again.

The most important thing to do is forgive yourself. You are not a terrible or lazy person. You are learning something new. Take the setback as a learning experience and move on. Next, make any needed changes as indicated by what caused the setback. Be analytical, not critical. Finally, get over it and move on. The past is no longer something you can control or change; so do not let it do anything else but serve as a learning tool. Take the day you have and make the most of it.

NO NUTS ALLOWED!

When starting something new, there is always the urge to go nuts and jump in with both feet. Use that excitement constructively. Focus it on starting your program properly and slowly. Avoid injuries and discouragement by starting at the proper level. Do not push yourself farther than you can go. Slow and steady may not be exciting, but it is effective. In addition to being fit, you will also be an expert at your exercise of choice.

"Ambition is a poor excuse for not having sense enough to be lazy."
—Charlie McCarthy

EXCUSES, EXCUSES, OR: AMBITION AMMUNITION

What do you think is the most frequent question asked of a personal trainer? It's probably not all that surprising that it has something to do with losing fat or shaping butts and thighs. What is truly sad is that you already know the best way to lose fat, don't you? You can ask any fitness expert how to lose fat all day long and you know what? The answer is going to be the same every time. Want to know what it is? "Quit making excuses!" Okay, it's not quite that simple, so keep reading.

STOP EATING

DONUTS

It may seem obvious, but sometimes people need to read it in plain black and white. Eighty percent of the results you get from your weight-loss routine come from what you eat. (Why do you think this book has such a big section on eating?) Can't get any clearer than that, right? So, your first step in any kind of weight-loss program should be to take a nice long look at what you're eating. Okay, it's scary. You must face this task with iron resolve (plastic will do). Here are a few basics:

• Pick up a journal. A blank one, silly. This journal will be your new best friend. In it, you will write down *every single thing* you eat each and every day for seven whole days. Don't try to change anything—just keep track of what and how much you're eating.

• After your seven days have elapsed, go through your journal and objectively (no shameful feelings allowed) decide what is your worst eating or drinking habit. Is it too much Coke? Is it eating one cinnamon roll per mile every morning on the way to work? Whatever it is, that's where you start. Vow to change that one habit and leave the rest of your eating alone. (Now it's one cinnamon roll every two miles.) Once you conquer that bad habit, move on to the next. Yes, this is gonna take a while—hey, do you want lifelong changes or instant gratification?

Muscle Myth
Exercising makes you tired.

Triceps Truth
Most people feel that exercising gives them even more energy than before. Regular exercise can also relieve stress.

GET YOUR LAZY ASS OFF THE COUCH

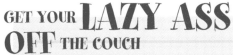

You know that you have to exercise. You know it, and yet you don't do it. Why? What is so terribly, horribly *wrong* with exercise, huh? You think it sucks don't you? How do you know if you don't do it consistently enough to get used to it? So, here's what you do: Right now—okay—or after you finish reading this, get off the chair, turn off your computer, and take a walk up the stairs, down the driveway, up the street, wherever. Just walk somewhere. Even if it's just for five minutes. Even if you get out of breath just getting up. *Do something!* There's a world out there, and you're missing it.

Okay, realistically, you need to be doing 30 to 45 minutes of cardio (and that means real cardio, like brisk walking, running, aerobics, swimming, etc.) four to five days a week if you want to lose weight. (Going to check the mail doesn't count.) But, you must be patient and start slowly. If you work too hard the first time, you'll hate it and then you may just quit. If you hate the exercise you're doing, how long do you think you'll stick with it? Probably not very long. Find something you like (or at least can tolerate) and go to it.

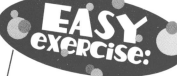

EASY exercise: knee Raise

Sit on a flat bench and support your body weight on your hands resting just behind you. Lean back slightly and straighten your legs into the air out in front of you. Bend your knees and pull them toward your chest. Return to the starting position. Repeat.

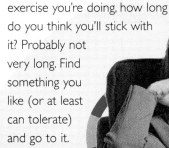

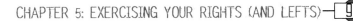

DISCOVER YOUR LEAN BODY TISSUE

Now that you've looked at your diet and pumped up your workouts, pick up a couple of weights and start building some muscle. Muscle burns more calories than fat and it also *takes up less space*, so the more you have, the more compact and stronger you are.

Plus, there's no better way to boost your metabolism. If you're just starting out, please find a personal trainer to help you out. Otherwise, you may end up wandering the free weight area forever with no clue how to escape. It's critical that you work each muscle group in the correct way since wasting time is not an option.

"I have never taken any exercise except sleeping and resting."
—Mark Twain

THE BOTTOM LINE

A combination of cardio, weight training, and a healthy diet is the only healthy and permanent way to lose body fat.

Starving yourself or working out until you collapse from cardiac distress is simply uncool and, in the long run, will only cause you to add even more flab to the old thighs. So get moving.

BEST MOVIES TO WATCH BEFORE WORKING OUT

- Rocky (Pick one!)
- Flashdance
- Staying Alive
- Fight Club
- Vision Quest
- Chariots of Fire
- Prefontaine
- Over the Top
- 10
- The Karate Kid

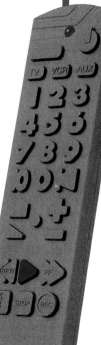

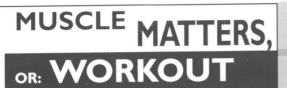

MUSCLE MATTERS, OR: WORKOUT WISDOM

When was the last time you looked in the mirror and thought to yourself, "Gee, I'm just way too toned and firm-looking." This has probably never happened, because muscle is the most magnificent stuff in our human bodies, and most people don't have enough of it! A simple strength training routine is all you need to treat your magnificent muscles like they matter!

Many of us have allowed our muscles to atrophy to a pitiful state; unused muscle fibers weaken and shrink until they are actually dormant. Dormant muscles are not in any condition to come to your rescue when you call on them, so injuries are far more likely. Muscle has many functions, and a toned, strong body is simply a delightful side effect.

A lot of people don't know this, but although muscles are devastatingly attractive, they are also your body's fat-burning mechanisms! The bigger and stronger your muscles, the more calories you burn on an hourly basis, at rest and at play. Studies have shown that strength trainers burn up to 100 calories more an hour during aerobic exercise than couch potatoes.

Don't you love it? The fitter you get, the more calories you burn an hour, and the easier it becomes to stay fit. Maintaining muscles requires more calories than maintaining fat stores—duh—so the more muscular you get, the higher your metabolic rate becomes. Other ways muscles help you that you may not know:

• By training your muscles, you also increase the strength of your bones and connective tissue (the tendons and ligaments), thus decreasing the risk of injury. When you strength train, the increasing muscle mass stimulates the bone to increase in density!

• Most adults lose about one-half pound of muscle per year after the age of twenty, mostly due to decreased activity!

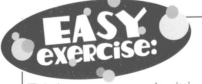

EASY exercise: ankle PUMPS

This is one you can do sitting down in a chair. With your feet planted firmly on the floor, pump both ankles up and down several times. This improves the circulation in your legs and tones the muscles in your lower leg.

• As your general strength increases, the effort required to perform daily routines (carrying groceries, working in the garden, brushing your hair, pouring milk) will be less taxing.

Don't neglect your valuable muscles! If you cut back on your calories and engage in aerobic exercise regularly (but not strength training), in the hopes of losing fat, your body is biologically obligated to enter "starvation mode." It becomes very reluctant to burn any fat stores because they are supposed to be for emergencies! Instead, your body will eat up muscle to power your exercise—unless you do something to build your muscles and keep them awake!

Traditionally, men have been the ones to concentrate on the condition of their muscles. In the olden days, before we walked entirely upright, males who were biggest and strongest got the best and most fertile females—just like in high school! The reality is that the modern man doesn't have to be the biggest and the strongest anymore; some of them just get off on it. Despite history, women are beginning to realize that they, too, can be dynamic, muscular, and above all, strong! You don't need to have bulging biceps or gross veins sticking out of your neck—only healthy, active muscles! How does one approach this most effectively? Here's a start.

EFFICIENT, EFFECTIVE STRENGTH TRAINING

Always warm up before lifting weights. Warming up reminds your muscles that they are about to be called into action! A good way to warm up is a brisk, 10-minute walk, or lifting very light weights a number of times. Now you're ready to pump iron! Put on some hyper music and get busy! Each lift of the weight is called a repetition, or rep, while a number of reps constitutes a set. Make sure you're lifting enough to challenge your muscles and build them up; you should find 12 reps challenging, and a second set downright difficult. If you don't challenge your muscles adequately, they will not understand the need to increase in size, and all your effort will be for nothing! Bummer.

Part of efficient strength training is working your muscles to failure. Lifting until your muscles actually fail is the best way to build definition! The failure of the muscle signals it that more fibers are necessary to perform this task next time.

After a short period of time, you will probably need to go up

EASY exercise: LATERAL CRUNCH

Lie on your right side with both legs bent so your thighs are at a 90 degree angle to your body. Extend your right arm on the floor, straight overhead. Place your left hand behind your head and point your elbow toward the ceiling. Slowly lift your rib cage toward your hip. Do not pull your elbow down, and try not to press on the floor with the right arm.

a weight to continue to challenge your muscles. Working through the burn, or beyond the point your muscles fail, is pointless. The signal has been received. Whether you reach failure after 8 reps or 80, the results are the same, so listen to your body instead of watching the clock or counting reps.

EASY exercise: SITTING BULL

This is one you can do sitting down. First, tighten your buttocks. Hold for the count of ten. Relax. Repeat several times. This helps prevent lower backache and fatigue in sitting.

CONSISTENCY

Strength training two to three times a week is really all you need to build healthy muscles! After lifting weights, the stiffness you feel, the burn you experience, is actually lactic acid that has built up in your muscles. Muscle tissue metabolizes sugar and carbohydrates to function, and lactic acid is a by-product of this. You need at least a day in between workouts to allow your muscles to recover from these challenges.

Working out sporadically will not get you the muscles you want. In fact, it takes three times as long to build muscle as it does to lose it, so any gains you have made in three weeks can actually be lost in as little as one week. Strength train to a video, or go to the gym, to be sure you are working all possible muscle groups, head to toe and front to back. A single missed muscle group can greatly decrease the effectiveness of your overall program.

STRETCH-ING

Never, ever lift weights without stretching before and immediately after your workout. Stretching your major muscle groups is essential to any exercise program, and to your physical health, particularly since tight muscles can cause you to exercise and move incorrectly by shifting body weight and motion to other muscles. Stretching helps muscles relax and increase their range of motion. Also, stretching can lengthen the muscles and prevent them from becoming bulky. By stretching after each exercise, and not waiting until the end of your session, you encourage the muscle to grow at a faster rate. Stretching also lessens any white-hot agony you may feel the next day as a result of your increased activity! Improper stretching, or not stretching at all, can lead to pulled muscles, soreness, and low performance levels, not to mention decreased flexibility. Stretch slowly, in a controlled way (no bobbing!), and hold each stretch for at least 20 seconds—the longer the better! Yoga is actually stretching exercises; the positions are simply held for minutes rather than seconds. Your stretch should be relaxed, accompanied by deep breathing, and should never hurt in any way. The old adage "no pain, no gain," is actually a load of crap! If it hurts, don't do it, especially when the pain is in your joints.

SORRY! THAT'S JUST THE WAY IT IS

Whatever muscle tissue you were born with is just how much you have. You can't increase the tissue itself, only its size! Women like Chyna of the WWF or men like Arnold you-know-who were born with a lot of muscle tissue—a lot more than the average homo sapien! They have worked very hard to increase the size of their muscle fibers, harder than most people would want to work, because they are huge bodybuilders who get huge results. You could be Chyna's workout buddy and probably never build muscles like hers!

Eating more protein will not build your muscles. For that, you have to work; you must stimulate your muscles and convince them that they're needed and valuable. There's just no way around it—you actually have to move your body! Think how hard that would be if you had no muscles!

Then think how hard *you* could be if you treat your muscles like they matter!

DAILY ACTIVITIES

Daily activities burn more calories than you might imagine. If you become a little more active in your daily life, you're on the way to losing weight.

ACTIVITY	CALORIES BURNED PER HOUR
• Sitting, watching TV	100
• Standing	140
• Making beds	155
• Housework	150-250
• Strolling	210
• Raking leaves	225
• Lawn-mowing (power)	250
• Lawn-mowing (push mower)	300-400
• Gardening	300-450

TRICEPS tip

To stave off hunger pangs and avoid bingeing because you're "starving," always keep a small snack handy, whether it be in your purse, backpack, filing cabinet, or pocket (front, that is). Individually wrapped crackers, hard candies, and even those tiny boxes of raisins could mean the difference between you getting home and making a sensible dinner and your stopping off at Magna Posterior Pizza on the way.

FAT OR FICTION,
OR: TRAINING MYTHS

There are so many myths associated with fat and exercise that they could almost fill their own book! One purpose of this book is to inform you about the incredible B.S. about diet, health, and fitness. These myths are not only misleading, they could actually be harmful. And they could contribute to the thousands of diet- and exercise-related deaths a year in the U.S. alone, which totally sucks.

Here are some of the myths circulating at present.

THE HARDER YOU WORK OUT, THE FASTER YOU'LL SEE THE EFFECTS

The truth is, the harder you work out, the faster you'll get hurt. Before you start killing yourself with a new exercise program, see a doctor. Or, at least, do some research first on the shape you're in (we cover that in Chapter 1, Mr. Speed Reader). Pushing yourself past a reasonable point, whether you're a veteran or a greenhorn, is less effective than pushing to that reasonable point and maintaining it. Low-intensity aerobic exercise over a longer period of time actually burns more fat than high-intensity exercise over a shorter period.

The "reasonable point" has no pain involved. Pain is a warning from your body that you're doing something harmful, so quit it. You should be breathing heavily enough that you can still speak, but not more than a sentence or two at a time. If your lungs are imploring you to slow down, and you can't shake a bout of nausea, you are past the reasonable point; you are hurting yourself for no reason. Plus, it's unlikely you'll stick to a tortuous routine as opposed to a simple and enjoyable one. If you hate jogging, don't jog. Swim, unless you hate swimming (yeah, we saw *Jaws* too), then bike. It only has to get you huffing and puffing comfortably. Yes, sex definitely counts.

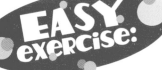

EASY exercise: TRICEPS DIPS

Sit down on a step platform, place your hands on either side of your thighs and grasp the edge of the step, fingers forward. Extend your legs out, then raise and lower yourself. The more your legs are bent, the easier the exercise is. If you don't have a step at home, you can use a chair (but don't let your shoulders go lower than your elbows, or you will not be supporting yourself enough).

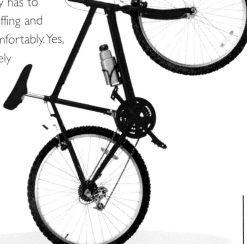

ACTIVITY	CALORIES BURNED PER HOUR
• Walking	300-420
• Bicycling	300-600
• Badminton	350
• Square dancing	350
• Bowling	400
• Leisurely swimming	260-750
• Brisk swimming	360-500
• Doubles tennis	360
• Singles tennis	480
• Volleyball (recreational)	300
• Light calisthenics	360
• Strenuous calisthenics	600
• Softball	280-400
• Golf	240-360
• Jogging	600-750
• Moderate running	870-1,020
• Sprinting	1,130-1,285
• Leisurely skating	420
• Fast skating	700
• Downhill skiing	500-600
• Cross-country skiing	560-1,020
• Basketball	360-660
• Rowing machine	840

SWEATING A LOT HAS SOMETHING TO DO WITH FITNESS

When all that salty sweat is running from your pores, it has only one function: to cool down your hot bod. Sweating a lot does not indicate you are in worse shape than anyone else, nor does it help you lose more weight. When your body loses moisture through sweat, you need to replace it and in a hurry. It's true that if you have ever stepped on a scale before and after a workout, you will notice a slight difference. This is lost moisture, however, not fat. As you approach improved fitness, you may sweat even more. Your body will adapt to your cooling and comfort needs in its usual efficient way.

LIGHT WEIGHTS ON YOUR ARMS OR LEGS BOOST YOUR WORKOUT

A fad emerged in the late 1980s that seemed to stick because it, on the surface, made sense. This fad involved small, handheld weights, or the kind that strapped around the ankles. You strap weights onto yourself before you head out the door for a walk or jog, and you somehow are combining strength and aerobic exercises. Strength training, however, requires heavy lifting for at least a dozen repetitions; carrying light weights around not only doesn't build muscle, it's hard on your joints. To increase your heart rate safely and more effectively, speed up whatever you're doing to a higher intensity. Pay close attention to your heart rate, listen to your body, and leave the tiny weights in the backyard for the resident garden gnomes.

EASY exercise: STANDING QUAD STRETCH

Stand on one leg and bring the heel of the other leg in toward your buttock. Keep your hips level, knees together, and supporting leg slightly bent. If you have trouble balancing, focus on something directly ahead of you or use a wall or chair for support.

CONTINUOUS EXERCISE IS MORE BENEFICIAL THAN INTERMITTENT

Whether you walk 45 minutes every morning, or 15 minutes three times a day, the benefits are the same. This can actually be easier to stick to, since 15 minutes throughout the day are easier to spare than 45 at a time. Another related myth is, unless you work out five times a week, an hour a day relentlessly, there is no point in exercising. Exercise helps even in small increments; a half hour walk three times a week can curb cravings, stress, and decrease the risk of high blood pressure and heart disease. Any tiny step toward regular exercise is better than none at all.

Moderation should always be your first instinct.

FAT MAKES YOU FAT

Glad you're sitting down for this one. This might come as a total shock, but fat is good for you! More than that, your body absolutely requires fat to function the way it should. Fatty acids can be obtained only by eating fat—your body does not produce them. Fatty acids are responsible for the control of your blood pressure, the clotting of your blood, and other useful inner-body type enterprises. Fat itself insulates, serves as an energy source, maintains healthy skin and hair, and aids in absorbing and transporting fat-soluble vitamins. Also, according to Brad Pitt, it makes kick-ass soap! (Or weren't you one of the dozen sick souls who saw *Fight Club*?) You ought to respect such a versatile substance; the problem with fat is that it has twice as many calories as anything else you eat: Nine calories to a carbohydrate's four!

Since weight is all about calories consumed versus calories burned, the more fat you eat, the more calories you consume, and the more energy you must expend to avoid gaining weight. It is possible to eat a low or even no-fat diet and still gain weight. It's the calories. End of story.

EASY exercise: squats

Put your hands straight out in front of you, and bend down as if you are going to sit in a chair. Remember to keep your legs hip-width apart, in order to make your balance steady. Do three sets of eight repetitions, with and without weights.

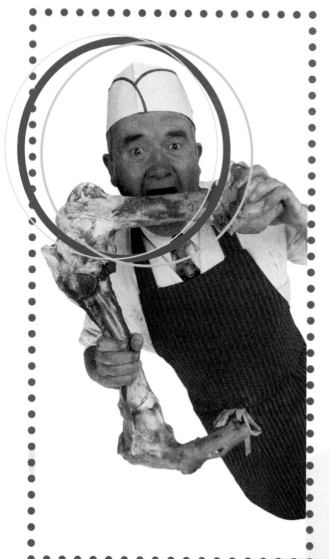

WHEN LOSING WEIGHT, YOU SHOULD BE HUNGRY ALL THE TIME

Feeling hungry all the time makes you feel cranky and deprived; this is because your body has no idea why you won't feed it. At the height of this crankiness, you will start to crave the quick energy afforded by high-sugar and high-fat snacks. Instead, eat a moderate amount of low-fat, low-calorie munchies when you've got the growlies. Grains, nuts, fruits—there are many foods you can turn to when you are hungry. Water can also be your best friend when your tummy feels empty between eating times; it's a natural appetite suppressant. Despite widespread belief, you can lose weight without suffering from constant hunger, and you will keep the weight off because you have set a long-term goal. Instead of lowering your metabolism to conserve calories, your body will start a continuous burn, since it isn't worried about the next influx of fuel. Remember, if your body is happy, so are you, theoretically.

EATING PROTEIN WILL MAKE YOU STRONG AND BUILD MORE MUSCLE

The only way to get strong is to strength train; the only way to build more muscle is to provoke the muscle fibers into growing. Eating a high-protein diet is not advantageous; most people get an adequate supply from daily meals and snacks. Athletes often consume four to five times their daily requirement because of this long-lived myth, despite the medical evidence that a high protein diet can damage the kidneys or liver. Muscles can only strengthen and adapt when you challenge them to do so with regular increases in the weight you lift; no amount of extra protein will encourage them to grow.

TRICEPS tip

Take advantage of the "Free Trial Membership" coupons many gyms place in the local paper or other fitness sources. As long as there is no commitment or money down, these are cost-free ways to inspect a gym from the inside out before actually signing up for an often long-term commitment.

MUSCLE MYTHS, OR: TRUTH OR BAYER

Does muscle matter? You bet it does. Muscle is what gives your body its shape. It's the difference between fab and flab, between body confidence and body insecurity, between looking great on the beach and wanting to disappear into a sand dune. Besides allowing you to look your best, there are some decided health advantages associated with packing a few pounds of lean beef onto your frame.

Consider, for example, the following:

• By strengthening sagging muscles you will be far less prone to that bane of the modern world—lower back problems.

• Your bones will be strengthened through the process of adding and shaping muscle. You will be a far less likely candidate for osteoporosis.

• You will have a lower resting blood pressure.

• Your gastrointestinal transit time will decrease. That puts you at a low risk of developing colon cancer.

• As you add muscle to your frame, you will be speeding up your metabolism, which naturally slows down after the age of thirty. You will be turning your body into an efficient fat burning furnace.

So, why are you still hesitating? You don't believe those crazy muscle myths that have been flying around do you? Not sure? Okay, lets set the record straight with a few choice myth busters.

(ENDORPHIN) RUSH HOUR

Recent studies have shown that people who exercise regularly are better able to deal with stress, both physical and mental, than those who don't. Exercise has also been shown to remedy anxiety and depression while at the same time actually elevating moods. Why? Your body has the ability to produce natural opiates or morphine-like chemicals on its own. When they are released in the brain, they inhabit cells that deal with pain, behavior, pleasure, and even emotions. During aerobic exercise, your pituitary gland releases more of one of these agents called beta endorphin. The resulting "exercise high" has been traced to more of this chemical traveling through your bloodstream in post-exercise tests.

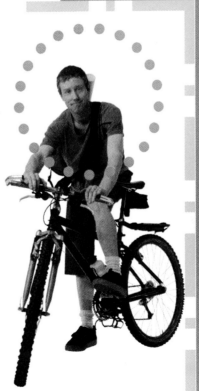

Exercisers often refer to this phenomena as a euphoric feeling or a "runner's high." Therefore, exercising aerobically not only benefits your heart and lung system, but it gives your brain a workout, too! The blood flow to your brain increases up to one-third more than at resting states. Exercise can also stimulate creativity by creating an alpha or relaxing state in your brain-wave activity, so creative blocks or even bad moods can be wiped away simply by taking a half-hour spin on your bike!

Myth No. 1—Women Will Lose Their Femininity

It is important to understand that a woman will not respond to weight training the same way a man does. It's a hormonal thing. To get big muscles you need testosterone—lots of it. Women just haven't got it in the same quantity as guys do. Unless a woman chooses to artificially boost her testosterone levels, she will not develop huge biceps, a thick neck, a husky voice, or any other male traits. (Like leaving the toilet seat up, for instance.) She will, however, accent her femininity by developing her womanly shape and tone while eliminating unsightly fat.

Myth No. 2—Muscle Can Turn into Fat

This one is a real no-brainer. But still it abounds. After you stop working out with weights, the theory goes, all of that hard earned beef will start to sag and will miraculously dissolve into dreadful, unsightly flab. Ugh! Happily, this one is way off target. Muscle is muscle, and fat is fat. You'll have better luck turning water into wine than converting muscle into fat. Of course, if a person slows down in his exercise routine, expends fewer calories, and increases his junk food intake, they'll get fatter. Their muscles will also atrophy slightly as a result of no longer being stressed. But it's still like comparing apples and oranges.

If you want to see a good example of what can happen to someone after they cut back on their workouts, check out Arnold Schwarzenegger's physique. Arnie retired from competitive bodybuilding in 1975. Today he is nowhere near the size he was back then, but—hey—we should all be so lucky as to have a physique like his in our late seventies or however old he is, right?

Myth No. 3—You Will Become Muscle Bound

"Sure, those muscles might look good, but I bet that guy can't really scratch himself."

You've probably heard similar comments about bodybuilders. You may have even thought that way yourself. Well, it's time to get enlightened. Lack of flexibility actually has nothing to do with an increase in muscle size and strength. It is the couch potato whose only exercise comes from stretching for the remote who needs to worry about losing flexibility, not the guys who are pushing weights.

In fact, properly executed weight training exercises have the added benefit of actually increasing flexibility as a result of exercising a muscle group through its full range of motion. And don't worry about those bodybuilders. Tom Platz, the guy with the absolute most muscular legs of all time, performs splits with ease and has been clocked in the 100-meter dash at a highly respectable 12 seconds. Not bad for a guy whose thighs measure 32 inches.

Myth No. 4—It's Easy to Get Injured Lifting Weights

Anything is dangerous if you don't do it properly. Working out with weights is certainly no exception. But what if you do it properly and follow sensible safety practices? Well, studies actually reveal that weight training injuries are significantly fewer per participation hour than for the majority of other sports and recreation activities. Muscle building and toning through weight training, then, is a very safe activity—provided that you follow the rules and don't get carried away trying to lift more weight than you are ready for.

Myth No.5— More Is Better

If three sets are good, then five has got to be great. If a 20-minute workout is productive, then a 40-minute one is going to double your results. It's simply a matter of logic. More is better, right? Well, that may work in the "greed is good" world of corporate warfare (as well it should), but when it comes to working out, forget it. Nothing will stop your progress like overtraining. In fact, the majority of people working out in gyms are actually doing more weight training than they should. A workout shouldn't be a mega-marathon endurance session. It should, rather, be a short and intense period of controlled exercise that takes your muscles to the point of max stimulation and then stops.

Going beyond this point will actually be counterproductive. Your muscles will become smaller and weaker rather than bigger and stronger. Once you've worked a muscle group, you need to give it enough time to recover—48 hours minimum. Work it again within this time frame and you will again be simply spinning your wheels. So, remember—get in, hit it hard, then get out and stay out until your body is rested enough to go at it again. Simple, ain't it?

MORE ENDORPHIN FACTS

• Endorphins have always existed in the human body, but were not identified until the mid-1970s.

• The average result of an exercise session is a euphoric or endorphin "high" for up to two hours after a workout.

• The word endorphin is abbreviated from "endogenous morphine," which means a morphine produced naturally in the body.

• It has been confirmed that endorphins have both neurological and spinal effects.

• Twenty different types of endorphins have been discovered in the nervous system.

• The most effective beta endorphin, which gives the most euphoric effect in the brain, is made up of 31 amino acids.

EASY exercise: BICEP CURLS WITH WEIGHTS

Stand with your feet hip-width apart for better balance, and slowly squeeze your right arm up to your chest, then lower it again. If you do not have any weights, you can use everyday household objects such as bags of sugar. Do eight repetitions, then move onto your left arm.

6
CALORIE CONFUSION

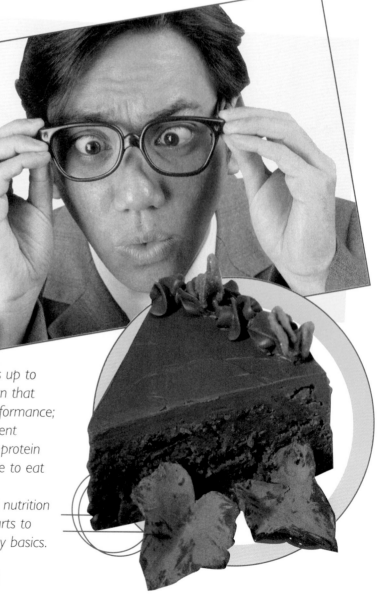

While you may not find an exercise called "Calorie Counting" in most fitness books, food and exercise go hand in hand. (Just like burgers and fries. Whoops, wrong diet.) The endorphin rush, the lower blood pressure, the increased stamina, the stronger muscles, they all tend to make fitness buffs and buffettes (not buffets, silly) more aware of what they put inside their bodies.

After all, a two-hour workout followed by a round of German chocolate cake is an equation that adds up to heft, not health. Of course, it's well known that some foods actually increase fitness performance; potassium-loaded bananas help to prevent cramps, for instance. Carbo-loading and protein pounding aside, it just makes good sense to eat better to feel better.

And while the subject of health and nutrition could fill another entire book, it never hurts to refresh yourself with a few of the healthy basics.

CONSTANT CRAVINGS:
THERE'S A DIFFERENCE BETWEEN BEING PLAIN OLD HUNGRY & MINDLESSLY CRAVING FOOD

How hungry do you allow yourself to become before you finally head for the refrigerator? Do you see your hunger as an irritating, whining kid who you shut up by gobbling an energy bar or grabbing a burger during your hectic day? Or maybe you're a slave to hunger. It strictly dictates when and why you eat, you wimp.

Don't you think it's a bit bizarre that you are being dominated by a simple biological signal? Are you, or are you not, the master of your own desires? Okay, you're definitely not. But why is our hunger so difficult to conquer?

The problem is that the signal is hard to interpret, because there are different degrees of hunger. We know we are hungry, but not what we are hungry for. And often, the hunger we feel isn't even for food.

Being hungry is not the same as craving food. Craving is caused by an emotional response, and not necessarily one related to food, either. Okay, it's confusing: Time of day, advertisements, habits—all can contribute to food cravings. There are four questions you should ask when you find yourself in the kitchen— you may discover that you are not hungry after all, but that your brain is instead responding to something external:

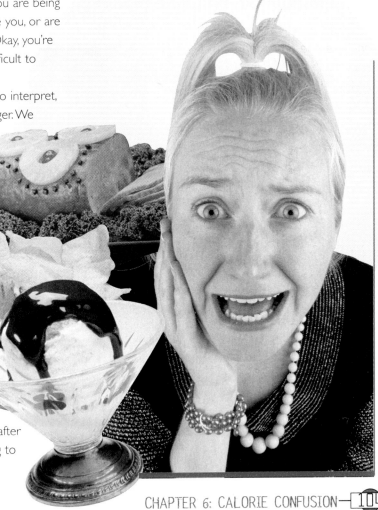

• When did I eat last?
• What am I craving?
• Am I actually hungry or has my appetite been temporarily stimulated?
• What is my reason for wanting to eat?

Never skip meals. By skipping a meal, you allow yourself to become overly hungry. Your blood sugar drops after about five hours, and your brain really doesn't care what you eat to raise it up again. The hungrier you are, the less likely you are to make sensible food choices. You allow the hunger to control you.

Instead of grabbing a meal here and there, try to eat every four or five hours. When your eating pattern is disordered, your brain is constantly anxious about where the next nourishment is coming from, sort of like an annoying date: "Are we going to eat, or what?" It

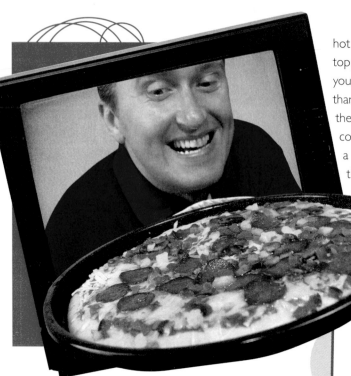

hot pizza, laden with all eight of your favorite meat toppings. Your brain recognizes these foods as some of your favorites, and just assumes you'll be having some, thank you very much. It preps you to eat, right down to the growling stomach and watering mouth. How convenient: You're hungry, and the pizza joint is having a "buy one slice get one free day." This is what makes these commercials so effective; their makers are quite aware of what they do to your brain. Pavlov and his dogs would be proud.

Make certain that it's actually hunger causing you to eat, and not stress or boredom. Regular exercise is an sends you repeated signals to be sure you remember to eat. It's always a good idea to eat a balanced diet, so the brain is wanting for nothing, and doesn't have an excuse to trigger a craving. When you're not ravenous or famished, but merely hungry, it's far more likely you'll think for a minute and reach for something reasonable like veggies, yogurt, milk, and other healthy snacks to satisfy that little gnawing. (Or a couple of Twinkies, whatever.)

Cravings take about 20 minutes to build, crest, and subside. Isn't it weird how we only seem to get cravings for junk food? How often does it strike you that, "Wow, I just suddenly want a dozen carrot sticks?" Try distracting yourself if you feel a food urge that isn't real hunger—go for a walk, read a book, make a call, murder the marketing guy in the next cubicle, whatever. If you find you're still craving at the end of the 20 minutes, go ahead: enjoy a rational portion. Most likely, however, you will be able to overcome the 20-minute craving.

Your senses can also betray you. Beware of food cues maliciously set by advertising bombardments. Food cues are sights, sounds, smells, or other external stimuli that crank up your cravings. It could be the rich, buttery smell of popcorn, or an appealing TV ad selling gooey,

LEAST FATTENING JUNK FOOD

- Baked potato chips
- Jelly beans
- Frozen yogurt
- Oatmeal cookies
- Popcorn
- Jell-O
- Pudding
- Graham crackers
- Fig Newtons
- Jujyfruits
- Fudgsicles
- Fruit popsicles

excellent stress release. Also, when we exercise aerobically, our brains release chemicals that make us feel good. It's probable your brain also releases these chemicals when you overindulge in your favorite foods, but eating a whole banana cream pie is not exactly riding your bike for 10 miles. The groovy, feel-good chemicals fade quickly, and if your route has been the Tour de Cream Pie, you are worse for the experience.

If your problem is not cravings at all, and you feel you're hungry all the time, the solution is simple: Eat. Deprivation is no way to live, and hunger is not a happy sensation. Just eat the right things (basically stuff that you'd feed to squirrels, rabbits, pigeons, or monkeys): nuts and seeds, fruit, raw vegetables, low-fat popcorn, pretzels. You can eat almost all day long, if you choose the right foods and eat reasonable portions. Cows call it grazing.

And don't forget water; it fills you up quite adequately if you drink eight glasses a day or so. Enjoy better skin, more energy, and less fatigue as a side effect of actually being properly hydrated for once. Sometimes your brain makes you think you're hungry, but truly, you need water, not food. Conscious eating doesn't mean you have to relinquish your beloved almond mocha fudge. It only means you'll appreciate it more when you enjoy it once or twice a week instead of daily at ten, two, and four.

So the way to consider hunger is not as an adversary or a wild beast or a whining kid. Hunger is the yellow light at an intersection: Everyone recognizes what it means, but not many people heed it or even think twice before running it. Hunger is a natural function of your body, and a valuable one—you'd be dead without it.

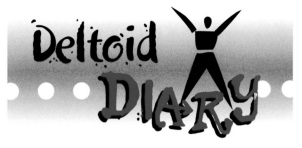

Jiggler's Journal

Climb aboard the triglyceride train and ride the Ring Ding roller coaster of two weeks of an average dieter's downhill life:

DAY 1

This is it! This is the big day! Today I will begin my new life. My new, thin life. I will succeed this time. I will stick to my diet. I will exercise every day. I will become a beautiful, thin, gorgeous, amazing woman. I am strong, and I know I can do it this time.

DAY 2

I am so proud of myself. All I ate today was a salad at lunch (no dressing) and some crackers. I stopped at the gym on my way home from work and spent 20 minutes on the stair machine, 20 minutes on weight training, and 20 minutes on the treadmill. I can do this!

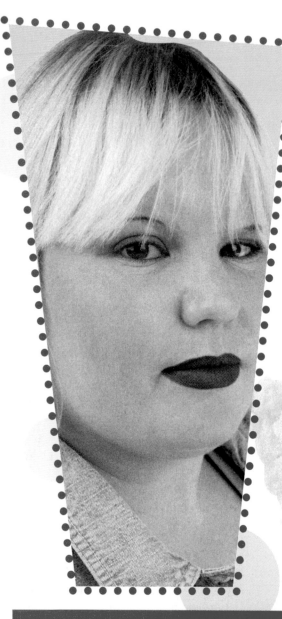

DAY 3

Couldn't work out today. Hell, I could barely walk today. Note to self: Don't overdo it. I'll feel better tomorrow. Oh, yeah, still sticking to my "salad only" deal. I'm really starting to think I can do this!

DAY 4

Feel a little better today; made it to the gym, but only as far as the juice bar. Had a carrot smoothie; that makes up for not working out, right? I had salad for lunch and dinner but couldn't resist a donut at work this morning (it was my morning to buy them). I'm not too worried, though, I'm sure I'll do better tomorrow. I mean, one slipup doesn't mean I've failed—does it?

"C is for cookie, it's good enough for me."

—Cookie Monster

DAY 5

Back on track! Spent 10 minutes on the stair machine, 10 minutes on weights, and 10 minutes on the treadmill. Had salad for lunch and dinner! I feel great! Does life get any better than this?

DAY 8

Missed a few days there—not much different though. Been stopping at the gym every day. What a great juice bar! The juice man there knows me by name. Kind of cute, too.

DAY 9

I slipped today and had a cookie—okay, so I had a whole bag of cookies, but I swear I'll work it off. I know I can do this. Just have to be strong.

DAY 10

Went to the gym to work out today, ended up at the juice bar again. (He is sooo cute!) I must be losing weight already because I think he was flirting with me. I spent so much time talking to him, I had to come home before I got to work out. Oh, well, I guess there's always tomorrow.

TRICEPS *tip*

Be realistic. Don't focus on exercises you find upleasant or uncomfortable. Choosing activities you enjoy will help you stick with your program. Plan for success.

DAY 12

Today I splurged at lunch—went to Luigi's. They make the most incredible shrimp scampi, gorgeous shrimp dripping in garlic butter sauce. Does life get any better than this?

DAY 14

Canceled my gym membership today. I don't really want to think about it, but maybe it will make me feel better. That quart of ice cream I just ate sure didn't help much.

Here is how my downfall began: I went to the gym today and headed for the juice bar (as usual). There was a group of people gathered around the bar, and they were all laughing. The bar is usually empty this time of day, so I asked one of the girls toward the back what was going on.

She tells me that Kevin (apparently that's the juice man's name) is telling this hysterically funny story about this fat chick who comes in like almost every day and hits on him—never works out, just drinks like four smoothies and chats him up.

At this point, she turns and actually looks at me. Of course, the second she

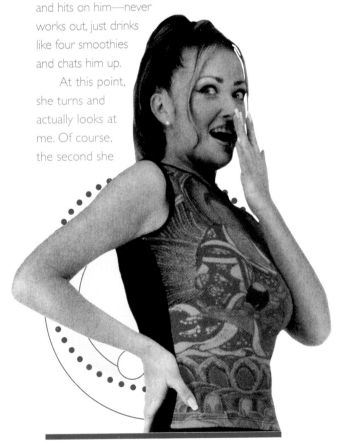

does she realizes that I must be the fat chick (how can you miss me?), which naturally sends her into gales of maniacal laughter, making everyone turn and look at me—and then they all lose it.

Why are people so cruel? I'm not giving up, though, as much as I want to. I'll just have to find another way.

DAY 16

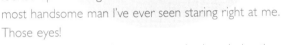

Was looking for a new gym today when I smelled this wonderful, sweet aroma wafting down the street. Following the smell, I found myself in the cutest little bakery, took a number, and waited. I looked up and caught the most handsome man I've ever seen staring right at me. Those eyes!

Anyway, it turned out we were both ordering the same thing: pumpernickel-rye loaf, two éclairs, and two napoleons. He asked me out on the spot. Told me he couldn't stop staring at me—I responded with an attitude, "Of course, how could you miss me?"

What he said next blew me away: "I agree! How could I miss those gorgeous eyes and drop dead legs? Now, how about that dinner?" Can you believe that? And dinner was great, he never once mentioned my weight and even forced me to share a dessert with him. We're going out again this weekend. Can this really be happening?

I've always thought I couldn't be happy unless I was thin, but does it really matter? Maybe it really is what's on the inside that counts. Maybe I should learn to appreciate myself for who I am—inside and out. For now though, I'm hungry. I think I'm gonna have an éclair—hell, you only live once right? I'll start looking for a new gym tomorrow!

PUZZLING PLATEAU

You rule. In the past few months, you've seen genuine progress; you've learned oodles about your body and what it needs to stay healthy. You've enjoyed compliments and twitters of envy from your friends and family. For the first time, buying clothes has been an enjoyable experience and when you look in the mirror, you're actually happy with what you see. Your body has never pleased you more nor maneuvered better, and you have only one and a half inches to go. After losing so much fat, it's hard to imagine yourself losing momentum; you are unstoppable, unshakeable, and unbreakable.

What the hell?

The fat is clinging to your body like a parasite. Your progress grinds to a halt, and though you are as unfailing as ever with your workouts, the fat remains. You feel discouraged, your motivation is failing, and you're kind of hacked off. What are you doing wrong?

Nothing. You're doing everything right. There are two possible explanations:

One is that you have reached your healthy weight. If you just can't seem to lose those last 10 pounds, your body may have made the decision for you, and stopped any further weight loss. Fitness is not about the scale or the last 10 pounds. It's about how you feel, how your clothes fit, and how long you can maintain your new level of fitness. If you are within ten pounds of your goal, it might be time to celebrate your new healthy body, and your new healthy future.

If you still have 20 or more pounds to lose, it's likely that you have achieved the notorious plateau. You may not like it, but you should at least be proud. A plateau is an indication that your body has adapted to your routine; it's a sign that you are fitter than you have ever been, and that your body considers your goal attained—that it has far less fat to lose than when you started this whole thing.

Damn frustrating, though, if you still have an inch and a half to go. To convince your body to adapt further, you need to make a few changes, known as plateau-busters.

DETERMINE THE CAUSE OF YOUR PLATEAU

Weight gain is the result of consuming more calories than you burn. The calories you consume are used to keep you alive—this is your Basic Metabolic Rate or BMR. As you lose weight, your body slows your metabolism because you need fewer calories for maintenance. Is it possible that those little calories have snuck up on you, settling into their little niches, and all because you need fewer calories now than ever before? Between your exercise and the exact eating pattern you have now, you have found the perfect stability to maintain your current weight. You are consuming exactly what you burn.

To lose weight, you must consume less than you burn. You either add activity to your exercise routine, or you eat fewer calories. Even minute changes can boost your metabolism enough to bust the plateau.

EXERCISE LONGER OR MORE OFTEN

Instead of your usual 30-minute walk, walk for 45 minutes. You don't even need to make this change for every day of the week. Adding a total of 30 or 45 minutes to your weekly routine will boost your BMR.

Adding a day to your weekly routine can boost your metabolism in the same way to burn more calories. Since you need to burn 3,500 calories to lose a pound of fat, the hotter your ovens are, the better. You could also stick to your current routine, but add a 20-minute walk or bike ride to the end of one or two days.

EXERCISE WITH GREATER INTENSITY

The easier your exercise gets, the less effective it becomes. Your body adapts to your demands, so of course you must continually demand more to keep it adapting. Try one-minute-long bursts of very high intensity exercise, followed by three or four minutes of exercise at your regular intensity. These sudden demands for energy send the metabolism into crazy overdrive; it even burns calories when you're lying on the couch watching reruns of *Magnum P. I.* Try to beat your own best time until you find your high intensity bursts are more frequent and even become lengthy.

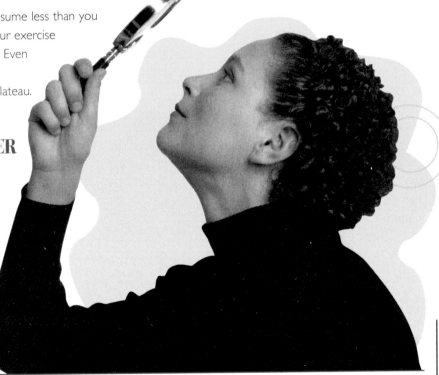

Remember, as your fitness level skyrockets, so will your metabolism, but you will need to continue to challenge yourself.

TRY DIFFERENT ACTIVITIES, ESPECIALLY WEIGHTS

Using different muscle groups in your exercise will encourage those muscles to grow, and so burn more calories. If you usually jog, reserve a couple of days in your routine for swimming; if you use the stair machine a lot, try kick boxing for a change. Variety can boost your BMR.

If you aren't already strength training, start now. Weightlifting two to three times a week will build strong, healthy muscles. Strong muscles are designed to burn fat: They are your fat-burning engines. The bigger they are, the more fat they burn at a faster rate. While a pound of fat needs a measly two calories for maintenance, a pound of muscle requires an amazing 35.

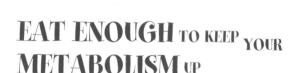

"Never eat more than you can lift."
—Miss Piggy

EAT ENOUGH TO KEEP YOUR METABOLISM UP

It is actually possible to over-reduce your caloric intake. If your body doesn't have enough calories to sustain your basic functions, between 1,000 and 3,000, it will crash your BMR right through the floor. People who eat breakfast have metabolisms 30 percent higher than breakfast fasters. Even with aerobic exercise and strength training, the BMR will remain in "starvation mode," burning as few calories as possible, and limiting energy as well as muscle production. You do need to limit your calories, but to a reasonable degree.

Eating foods like crunchy vegetables not only fills you up, but your body actually burns more calories in the process of digesting those celery sticks or summer squash than are contained in the foods themselves. Drink lots of water, too, to help keep you feeling full and hydrated.

If you're certain you've hit a plateau instead of reaching your healthy body weight, you must rediscover a most valuable virtue: patience. A pound a week may not seem very impressive, but it is about the rate you should expect, especially after overcoming a plateau and kicking its ass. Stay away from the scale—dispose of it altogether. Concentrate on how far you've come, not how far you have to go. Forget the bewilderment you felt during your plateau, and, even knowing you could land on another in the future, dread it less because you know the cause and the cures.

TOP-5 SIGNS YOU'VE HIT A DIETING PLATEAU

5.) "A whole week eating nothing but lard sandwiches and still 300 pounds. What the—"

4.) "Why haven't I lost any weight? I thought Snickers was less fattening than Butterfinger."

3.) "Honey, there's something wrong with the scale again."

2.) "So why do they call that guy in the Austin Powers sequel Fat Bastard?"

1.) Richard Simmons stops calling.

(LOSING THE) BATTLE OF THE BULGE, OR: WINNING THE WEIGHT WAR

Is there any other way to describe the endless struggle to keep the pounds off than to declare it a "battle?" In the pursuit of a healthy weight, dieters are armed with new and improved equipment for combat with cellulite and added pounds. The miracles of modern science have outfitted brave souls with high-tech instruments in order to face the confusion and despair surrounding the notion of the ideal body. The battle goes beyond the physical and attacks the mental state of seemingly normal people. To help you win your "battle of the bulge," however, we've included a few simple tips to beat those, in the words of k. d. lang, "constant cravings."

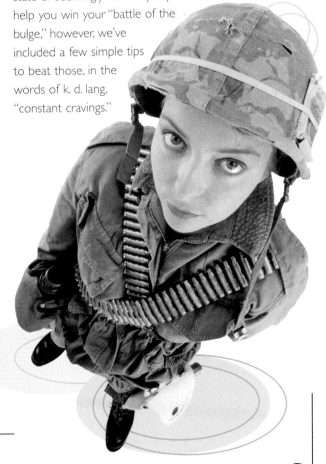

DRINK UNLEADED

The war over caffeine wages on. Is it addictive? Come on, do we really need a scientific survey to tell us that without our morning cup of java, we'd all be on a rooftop sniping strangers on the way to work in the morning? Do soda makers put caffeine in Coke to make us drink more? Duh! But how does it affect your diet?

In the old days, the belief was that having a can of soda to overcome your afternoon lull was better than having a snack. Okay, let's try out this hypothesis: It's 4 p.m., you're still an hour and a half away from clocking out, not to mention the 40 more minutes you'll spend in traffic. You haven't eaten since lunch, you still have a pile of paperwork to go through, so you can: a.) have a can of fat-free, sugar-free diet soda and try to survive on caffeine alone until you get home around 6; or you can: b.) stroll down to the break room and invest 75 cents in a cold cup of low-fat yogurt for about 200 calories and three grams of fat.

Hmm, instinct and savvy marketing tells us to go for the diet soda. It's quick, it's simple, and we all know that caffeine is the answer to everything. Okay, glug, glug, there you have it. Now you're fine for about half an hour, but your head is buzzing, your stomach is still empty, and not only that, you're feeling a little too high and the only thing that will even you out is something substantial in your stomach. So, what do you do? It's down to the vending machine anyway, where instead of buying that yogurt, your shaky cravings take over and you buy not one but two dangling packs of cheese or peanut butter crackers. Gulp, yum, yum, gulp. Now you're back to normal.

Sound familiar? Now let's try the yogurt scenario. Clomp, clomp, it's down to the break room for you. Spoon, yum, yum, spoon, and there you have it. Naturally, there's none of the caffeine rush, no instant euphoria. But there is a nice, filling sense of, well, being full. And what doesn't send you rocketing up surely won't send you spiraling down when the caffeine wears off.

"Even overweight cats instinctively know the cardinal rule: When fat, arrange yourself in slim poses."
—John Weitz, American designer

HEALTHY
WAYS TO CELEBRATE
WEIGHT LOSS

- Throw out ugly clothes that never fit before

- Burn the clothes in your closet that are now too big

- Buy a new outfit

- Get a makeover

- A weekend getaway to a spa

- Go out for drinks!

- Go out for a nice (but reasonably healthy) dinner

- Buy a skimpy bathing suit and saunter down the beach

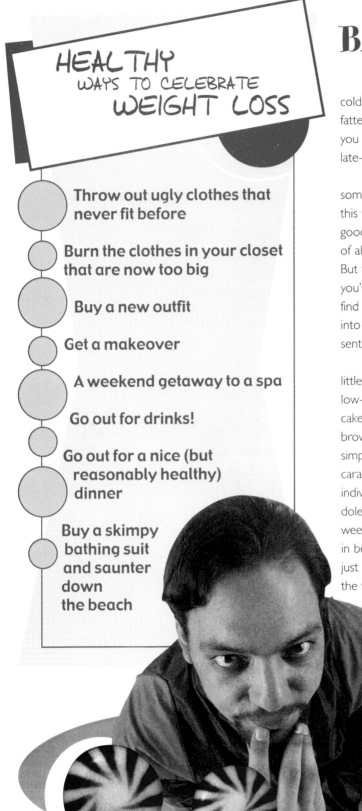

BABY STEPS

Another important tip is to remember not to go cold turkey. Starting a diet by tossing out every single fattening thing in the house is one sure way to drive you straight to the convenience store for a little late-night Ben & Jerry's love fest.

Yes, we all know it's more "dramatic" to say something like, "That's it, I'm through with sugar as of this very minute. Bye-bye Butterfinger, so long Snickers, good night, Mr. Goodbar." Followed by a trash can full of all that leftover Christmas, Easter, or Valentine's candy. But what's the inevitable second act? Five hours later you've downed every spare fortune cookie you can find in your soy sauce drawer, not to mention dived into that forgotten box of saltwater taffy Aunt Shirley sent you three years ago. ("Hey, not bad!")

So why not learn from your mistakes and leave a little candy around the house or office to avoid those low-sugar blues? Nothing wild and crazy, like a side of cake from the local bakery or a case of Little Debbie brownie's from Sam's Club. Just make it something simple and small, like hard candy or caramels. Make sure that they are individually wrapped, so that you can dole them out throughout the day, week, or even month. A Starlight Mint in between breakfast and lunch could just mean the difference between hitting the vending machine for a bag of miniature Oreos, or starving until lunch and wolfing at an all-you-can-eat buffet with the passion of White Fang.

Do-It-Yourself

There's no doubt that today's modern world offers us convenience everywhere we turn. From cell phones to e-mail, from take-out Chinese to Slurpees, it's all there, whenever we want it. Forgot to pack a lunch for work? Simply stop off at a

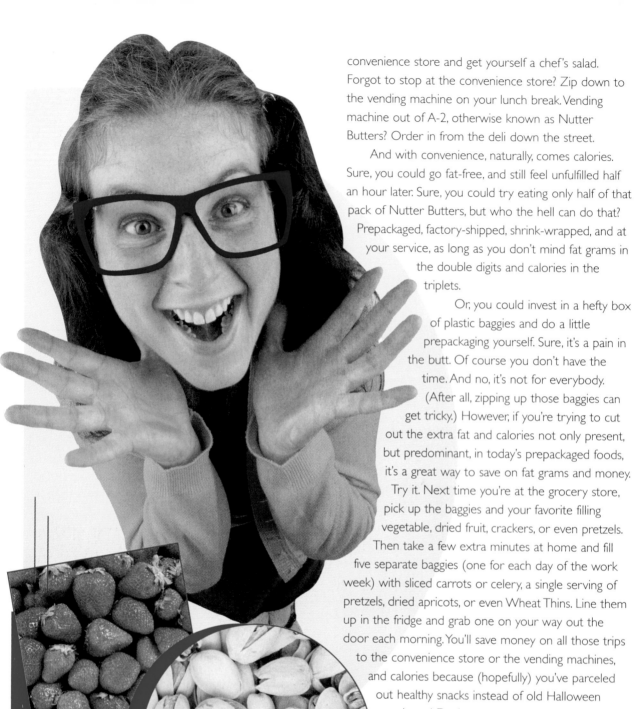

convenience store and get yourself a chef's salad. Forgot to stop at the convenience store? Zip down to the vending machine on your lunch break. Vending machine out of A-2, otherwise known as Nutter Butters? Order in from the deli down the street.

And with convenience, naturally, comes calories. Sure, you could go fat-free, and still feel unfulfilled half an hour later. Sure, you could try eating only half of that pack of Nutter Butters, but who the hell can do that? Prepackaged, factory-shipped, shrink-wrapped, and at your service, as long as you don't mind fat grams in the double digits and calories in the triplets.

Or, you could invest in a hefty box of plastic baggies and do a little prepackaging yourself. Sure, it's a pain in the butt. Of course you don't have the time. And no, it's not for everybody. (After all, zipping up those baggies can get tricky.) However, if you're trying to cut out the extra fat and calories not only present, but predominant, in today's prepackaged foods, it's a great way to save on fat grams and money. Try it. Next time you're at the grocery store, pick up the baggies and your favorite filling vegetable, dried fruit, crackers, or even pretzels. Then take a few extra minutes at home and fill five separate baggies (one for each day of the work week) with sliced carrots or celery, a single serving of pretzels, dried apricots, or even Wheat Thins. Line them up in the fridge and grab one on your way out the door each morning. You'll save money on all those trips to the convenience store or the vending machines, and calories because (hopefully) you've parceled out healthy snacks instead of old Halloween candy and Doritos.

When you get tired of a week's worth of pretzels or dried banana chips, it's time to up the ante and create a few combinations of your own. How about pretzel sticks and raisins? Or dried apricots and reduced fat peanuts? Or all four. Make a big batch of your calorie conscious concoctions and dole them out into five servings for a brand new week of snacking "fun."

TOMORROW NEVER DIE(T)S

Have you ever considered the possibility that diets don't work? You've heard this before, sure, but did you really believe it? Deep down, in your heart, in the pit of your stomach, do you really, truly believe that diets are a waste of time? It's not an easy thing to forget everything you have been taught by the world around you about eating. It's not an easy thing to relearn how to do something you thought you've known how to do for your entire life.

Believe it. You're going to have to relearn how to eat.

DIETS CAN BE DANGEROUS

In general, if you don't eat enough, your body worries you might be starving, so it slows its metabolic rate to conserve calories. If it's not getting enough calories to sustain functions, your body will break down muscle and other tissue for the energy it needs long before it will attack fat stores. Few diets take this into account or warn that exercise isn't just an option, it's a must. In other words, by going on a diet, you are actually slowing your metabolism and sabotaging your own efforts.

Despite the seemingly sensational success of their testimonials, diets that promise quick and easy weight loss are rarely balanced or nutritious. An unbalanced diet followed for a long period of time can be very damaging to your body. Any diet that recommends "no something" or "all something" could be characterized as unbalanced, sort of like your crazy uncle Chester. Would you take diet advice from him?

These diets are dreamed up by capitalists whose only concern, whose only lust in life, whose raison d'être, is to make money; they care not a whit about your health, happiness, prosperity, dog, or job. Don't you think you could sit down and invent a drastic diet, and for some reason it would work? Probably in about ten minutes. Would you follow it, though? Chances are, unless you're a doctor or a nutritionist, not bloody likely. Then why follow a diet laid out by some other bozo with a marketing machine behind him?

Consider these tell-tale tip-offs:

- Is there a promise of rapid weight loss?
- Is a single food the miraculous key?
- Does the diet eliminate one food (or one nutrient, like carbohydrates)?
- Are one or more of the five food groups on the basic food group pyramid eliminated?
- Does the diet require you to skip meals?
- Does the diet set a caloric limit below 1,000 calories a day (without constant medical supervision)?
- Does the diet have some product to sell (food you must buy)?

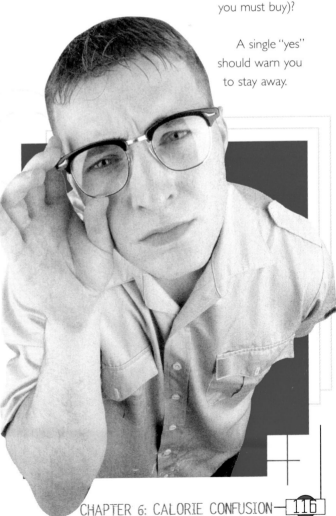

A single "yes" should warn you to stay away.

DIETS ARE A SHORT-TERM QUICK FIX

Researchers have found that speedy weight loss is usually followed by speedier weight gain, and may initiate eating disorders. Once the dieters are off the diet, lost and alone, they invariably fall back into their old eating habits. Despite the weeks of restriction, painstaking attention, and deprivation, results are maddeningly temporary.

Stupid diets. They don't teach you how to handle obstacles, what to do when backed into a corner by an aggressive triple fudge peanut butter cheesecake, or how to nourish your brain while you attend to your body. Diets whisper evils in your ear until you're sure that piece of cheesecake might be worth trading almost anything for. Diets set you up for failure, and dutifully knock you down. They blame you for pitfalls and convince you it's good and pleasurable to be hungry! Diets try to overrule the convictions your body was born with.

Nobody can restrict themselves to a diet for the rest of their lives. Nobody can drink a milkshake twice a day for the next 50 years. Nobody can eat cabbage soup for decades and decades. The key, as everyone seems to know but ignore, is a nutritionally balanced diet laden with vegetables, fruits, whole grains, fish, nuts, and other stuff your body cherishes and utilizes.

Monounsaturated fats, like olive oil, keep you from feeling hungry again just as quickly as less-healthy polyunsaturates such as vegetable oil. Small meals stretched over the whole day—large snacks, almost—are more likely to maintain your satisfaction, prevent you from overeating, and encourage your metabolism to burn, baby, burn!

Food is not the enemy, and it's time you stopped treating it as such. Eat smaller portions; your stomach doesn't know you're full for 20 minutes after eating. Be liberal with seasoning, spices, citrus, and herbs—if it tastes amazing, you won't need as much to feel satisfied. Also important is that your preferences and choices are a factor in the preparation of your food, putting the control back into your life. Do your homework—research your body, how it works, and how to take care of it. Be kind to yourself, enjoy every bite; it's not that hard. Believe it.

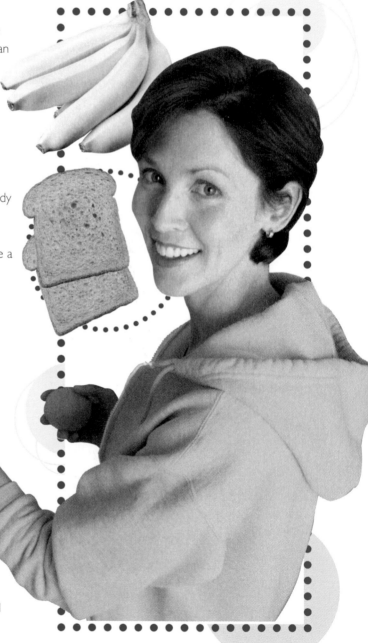

DIETS
MAKE YOU MISERABLE

Restricting food intake for the purposes of weight loss is known as a diet. Face it—restrictions are not something we humans do well with. It's doubtful you could name one single restriction that society has created that it has been able to accept and obey. Okay, stoplights. But restrictions make us unhappy, especially unreasonable ones! Diets are all about unreasonable restrictions and unreasonable expectations; is it any wonder they fail? You are so unhappy while on the diet that you can't wait to get off it! What the hell is the point of that?

Diets dictate what to eat and what not to eat, despite individual inclination; diets stir up a veritable cocktail of misery and woe, guilt, resentment, and disappointment. Sounds like fun, but maybe you should pass! The boredom! The hunger!

Boredom and hunger team up on a regular basis to kick your ass. Depriving yourself of the things you want to eat only makes you prone to stuffing your face when you finally snap. To make matters worse, when you're very hungry from a day of dieting, your body craves the most fatty, most readily available food within your field of vision, and it will take a Herculean effort not to cave in to your body's desires. Most people are not even capable of a Pee Wee Herman effort every day, especially on a continuing basis.

HUNGER PANGS,
OR: SNEAKY SNACKINGS

Should significant others and their partners or husband and wife diet together? When this particular couple opted to give it a try, their friends said they'd probably lost their minds. It seemed, however, to be the only way they could think of to motivate themselves to lose some weight.

A DIETER'S DIARY

They needed to shed a few pounds that had crept upon their late-twenties girths in recent years. Judy, although not a replica of Twiggy, was a beautiful woman. She had even been a fashion model during her youth. But now she could certainly afford to lose ten or twelve extra pounds, and her husband needed to lose about that much or more himself. They figured they had nothing to lose and everything to gain by joining efforts and cheering each other on. (Shouldn't it be everything to lose and nothing to gain—in terms of weight loss? Oh, well!)

Throughout the weekend they held a pep rally, encouraging each

"The second day of a diet is always easier than the first. By the second day you're off it."

—Jackie Gleason

other to lose the weight. They would begin dieting on the following Monday. When day one arrived it proceeded quite uneventfully. However, after drinking eight glasses of water apiece, and eating enough salad to satisfy a dozen rabbits, Judy and Kurt were positively squirming at the notion of visiting an ice cream shop and inhaling a hot fudge sundae.

One positive feature of their diet was that being one half of a dieting duo seemed to keep them both brutally honest. When the naughty cravings became too intense, they simply set their minds in a different direction and went to bed. (It is said that sex burns calories—there may be something to this dieting thing after all!)

Day two passed like a charm. Bless the creator of fat-free pudding cups! They staved off the typical hunger pangs as well as two killer chocolate cravings Judy suffered in the same hour. Kurt seemed to fare better than Judy did, as he genuinely enjoyed the stringy bitter grapefruit sections and tasteless carrot sticks.

By day three Judy felt certain she could fit back into a size 4, but of course that was merely an illusion. In reality, however, her size 10s were feeling far more comfortable than they had in months. (But was it the dieting or the sex that actually caused the weight loss?)

Day four found the dieting duo taking a walk at lunchtime, and indulging in a fresh fruit salad and fat-free frozen yogurt for dinner. By now they'd even managed to drink their numerous quarts of water without immediately running to the bathroom.

The fifth day brought a definite cause for celebration.

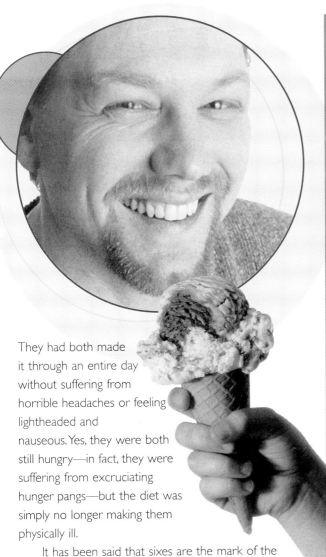

HEALTHY SNACKS

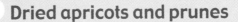

- Low-salt pretzels
- Hummus and pita bread
- Dried apricots and prunes
- Baked and barbecued chicken breasts
- Baked tortilla chips with bean dip
- Low-fat, low-salt ham
- Mozzarella string cheese
- Baked potato with salsa and yogurt
- Peanut butter on apple slices
- Graham crackers
- Baked, low-salt potato chips (single serving size)
- Yogurt or pudding popsicles
- Pasta salads

They had both made it through an entire day without suffering from horrible headaches or feeling lightheaded and nauseous. Yes, they were both still hungry—in fact, they were suffering from excruciating hunger pangs—but the diet was simply no longer making them physically ill.

It has been said that sixes are the mark of the devil, and that must be the reason why on day six the deprived couple cheated and indulged in double scoops of triple fudge walnut ice cream on crunchy sugar cones. After feeling horribly guilty and confessing their sins to their Creator, they learned of a whole new slew of illicit dieting faux pas, including indulgences of several Oreo cookies and two entire boxes of turtle candies. What conniving sneaks they had turned out to be!

TOP-5 SIGNS YOU'RE NOT QUITE READY TO WEIGH IN YET

5. "Just one more Twinkie, honey. PLEASE! What can it hurt?"

4. Your death grip on the refrigerator door.

3. "I just ran over the scale? How did that get under there?"

2. "Hey, these slippers weigh at least thirty pounds!"

1. "What do you mean I have to put both feet on?"

At the one-week mark came the much anticipated weigh-in. Kurt learned that he had successfully lost four pounds, which for only a week's worth of dieting was really quite a lot of weight. He had indeed accomplished some of what he'd set out to do. Judy lost a mere two and a half pounds, but seemed to be satisfied with those results. Both Judy and Kurt felt they were fully deserving of some type of reward for their dieting efforts. After all, they had yielded positive results. And they had endured a whole week's worth of hunger pangs.

So they headed, of course, to the nearest restaurant. After perusing the menu, they opted to indulge, not in the minute portions customary at this place, but with an item the kitchen couldn't cheat on: a pair of 10-ounce sirloin steaks, cooked to a perfect rare temperature. Beside each of their steaks, they insisted on every potato side dish available, and when the waiter sniffed whether they cared for salads, Kurt said they'd have the Mediterranean bobo-bean with lattice lettuce but the suggested dressing (piss-sour vinaigrette) wouldn't do. Lather on the blue cheese, waiter boy.

Retiring later that same evening, the satiated couple felt bloated, piggish, and downright lousy. In fact, they found themselves almost yearning for the dull ache of the hunger pangs. They would even be a welcome relief from the sick feeling they experienced since polishing off their enormous meals. After a restless night of fitful, sporadic shuteye, Kurt and Judy resolved to resume their diets, and vowed to adhere to the calorie counts and fat gram counts from that moment on.

A week later, and an additional three pounds for Kurt and two for Judy, the shrinking couple made their way back to the restaurant. They ordered an even bigger cut of fatty red meat and splurged with an appetizer this time, too. Toward the end of their feeding frenzy, they were approached by a familiar face. It turned out to be the woman who weighed them in each week at their diet center.

"Hi there," she said as she cheerfully approached their table.

Instantly feeling guilty for having been caught at their game, Kurt and Judy hung their heads low and prepared to explain away their deviation from the recommended diet.

The diet lady interrupted Kurt just as he was about to spill the beans.

"I was having the most terrible hunger pains," she began, "so I knew I'd have to treat myself to a nice dinner, and they'd go away. It happens every now and then—even to the best of long-term dieters."

Kurt and Judy breathed enormous sighs of relief. They weren't as bad as they were beginning to feel.

Smiling at the diet lady, Kurt extended his hand and invited her to sit down with them at their table. She happily obliged.

When the waiter returned, Kurt and Judy knew that there was no chance of sneaking the decadent dessert that was featured on tonight's menu. It's just as well. They'd already cheated and been caught. "Dessert this evening?" the waiter inquired.

"Oh, my goodness, no," Judy said.

"No room for it," Kurt said as he patted his belly in mock fullness. "We're not crossing that line."

"Madame?" the waiter asked the diet lady.

"Oh, yes, please," she answered. "I'd like a piece of your double chocolate fudge cake, with a scoop of vanilla ice cream on the side. On second thought, make it a double!"

Judy and Kurt looked at each other and then said in unison, "Well, now that you mention it—"

> *"I have a great diet. You're allowed to eat anything you want, but you must eat it with naked fat people."*
> —Ed Bluestone

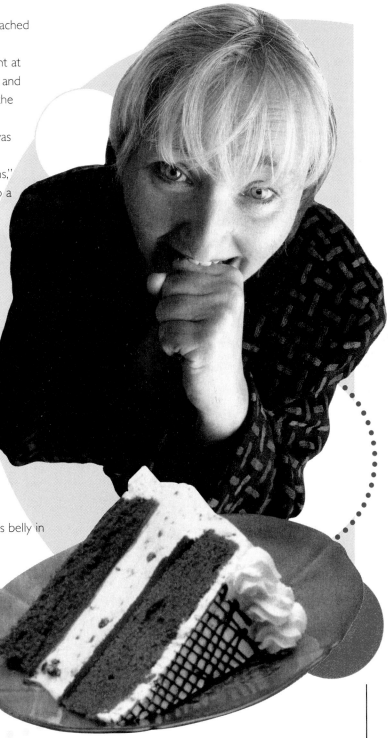

7
SEVEN
FITNESS
FADS

Considering that the dual industries of exercise and fitness generate profits that fall in the size XXXXXL category, it shouldn't be any surprise that medical quacks and exercise entrepreneurs alike come up with a bevy of bogus products, diets, gear, and equipment each year to satisfy our health lust.

From shady diets to faulty barbells, from helium-filled running shoes to invisible jump ropes (hey, you never miss), today's gadget grifters see a fast way to make a quick buck off of the modern American's obsession with physical perfection.

And it's not just the nameless and the faceless that pan for your muscle money each year. From Suzanne Somers's latest abdominal tightener to a dripping Richard Simmons *Sweatin' to the Oldies* to Chuck Norris gliding on some cable machine that seems about as substantial as his acting ability, celebrities are in on this cellulite cash cow as well.

So what's a poor body to do? Read on.

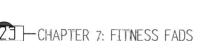

CREAMING YOUR "GENES," OR: LOTION POTION

If Ponce de Leon could have watched late night infomercials, he might not have bothered ever going to Florida in search of the fountain of youth or spring break or whatever he was looking for. He would have only had to pick up his phone and dial an 800 number to buy a bottle of youth elixir. These magical age-reducing, fat-melting concoctions flooding the market could have erased those "trouble areas" and given him the slim, vigorous, swashbuckling physique he dreamed of. At least, that's what the advertising and cosmetic companies would have us believe.

People like Ponce have been looking for a magic something—balms, pills, tonics, potions, or waters—since our ancestors started working out with bones and clubs. Just leaf through the literary canon. There's Tristan who guzzles love potions and Puck running around driving everyone mad with his impish tonic. And every child knows the archetypal witch, mixing hemlock, toad's head, and eye of newt in her bubbling vat. Sounds pretty disgusting, huh? Would you smear that concoction on your face?

Yet, cosmetic companies and fat melting creams use ingredients so mysterious and grotesque they would make Broom Hilda queasy. Their labels boast of turtle oil, shark oil, queen bee royal jelly, chick embryo extract, pigskin, and horse blood serum. And even if you did slim down, who is going to want to cuddle with somebody reeking of chick embryo?

The FDA actually has a name for these mysterious ingredients with the exotic names—"puffery." Puffery is a word for gimmick additives. For instance, eye of newt and pigskin are probably equally effective in shrinking all that cellulite on your thighs. The exotic name is no more than a canard to convince eager dieters that this new cream will turn toads into glamorous French runway models. The ingredients are so bizarre and disgusting that they must melt cellulite like microwaves melt butter.

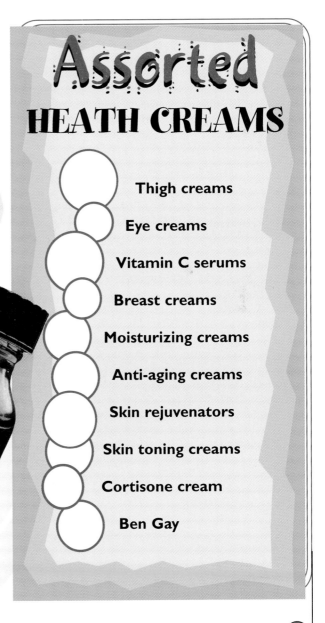

Assorted HEATH CREAMS

- Thigh creams
- Eye creams
- Vitamin C serums
- Breast creams
- Moisturizing creams
- Anti-aging creams
- Skin rejuvenators
- Skin toning creams
- Cortisone cream
- Ben Gay

I DIDN'T EVEN KNOW I Had Cellulite!

Try finding medical research on cellulite. You would have better luck finding Jimmy Hoffa. The word cellulite was created by advertising agencies, not the medical profession. In order to sell a product—say fat melting cream—you have to create a need for it. Most people weren't even aware they had cellulite until the advertising giants compared the thighs of an average woman to the air brushed thighs of super models like Cindy Crawford. Millions of women across the country were sure shocked one evening watching prime time with the family. And millions of husbands, you can bet, were up that night assuring their wives that their thighs were, "the most beautiful thighs in the world, honey buns, uh, sweetie."

What causes those fatty deposits on our thighs some advertising executive kindly named cellulite? Bad eating habits and stress are two primary causes. Spending less time in the drive-thru will shrink that cellulite faster than a jar of magical cream. It's not the fat causing the problem. The problem is all the garbage we feed ourselves in this high stress, manic world that keeps our fat cells from working properly.

FAT Is YOUR FRIEND

Fat cells are really bundles of stored energy. Who doesn't like energy? You can't do the Tour de France or even play a hand of poker without energy. Americans are in love with energy. Just look at all the power lines outside your home. How can we love energy, but hate fat? It's like adoring your car but hating gasoline. Fat should really be your friend, not your enemy.

Let's look at how fat helps you. It works like a warehouse storing up bundles of energy called lipids. Lipids are chiefly fats, phospholipids, and steroids. These bundles of lipids in our fat cells reserve energy, as mentioned above, and act as a cushion for our internal organs. Without fat all our internal organs would

bounce around like a bag of tomatoes every time we rode a roller coaster. One sudden stop in your car and your heart and liver would switch places.

Sometimes, however, excess fat produces "cottage-cheese" thighs. This is not caused by malicious fat cells conspiring to make you look like a hippopotamus for your birthday party. A discrepancy between the number of calories a person takes in and the amount of energy they use causes it. Fat cells will continue to store up lipids until they are used.

However, the sudden reduction of fat some miracle cures provide is only an illusion. The number of lipids in the fat cells will decrease, but the fat cells themselves rarely divide and are very long lived. As soon as a person starts consuming more calories than they burn in an average day, those fat cells will inflate again. This is what is called the "yo-yo effect."

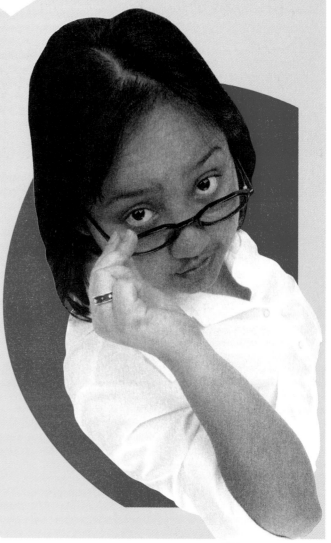

THE NEW
Puffery

The idea of toad skin in our cosmetics and diet supplements is laughable today. We think of ourselves as savvy and above the superstitious ingredients in witch's brew. Therefore, a good, strong scientific name is more comforting than a pinch of black cat dung. The shift in faith from the superstitious to the scientific hasn't escaped the companies marketing their fat burning creams.

Check out jars of fat melting cream, and you'll find the ingredient aminophyline. Wrap your mouth around that word—aminophyline. If it has five syllables, it must work! According to advertisements, this chemical is used for "spot reduction of fat." They mean that for best results you should place it on one "troubled area" at a time. It'll supposedly also "turn orange peel skin" into "peach smooth" skin. So, after applying this wonder balm, your bumpy thighs will turn into fuzzy thighs? Is that what they mean? It's a vision to consider.

What these advertisements fail to tell us is exactly what aminophyline is.

Aminophyline is an FDA approved drug used primarily in asthma medications. As a bronchodilator it's used to relax muscles when inhaled and to jump-start the body's metabolism. In other words, it's speed lite. In creams, aminophyline reduces fat by dehydrating the skin where it's applied. So, once a person drinks enough liquid or stops applying the ointment, the cellulite blossoms again. Already, this wonder drug is losing some of its luster.

There are also dangers when using aminophyline that advertisers fail to inform us of. The FDA is concerned about its use in creams because there is evidence some people can suffer allergic reactions to the chemical. They also strongly advise asthma patients to avoid these creams since there's a possibility they could develop an allergy to aminophyline that would compromise their treatment. Imagine becoming allergic to your own medication.

Aminophyline can also irritate the nervous system, cause seizures, and contribute to heart arrhythmia. So, a person wishing to try one of these creams after all this should still consult her physician, especially if she's having any health problems. These creams are not just harmless cosmetics as many companies would like us to believe. According to the Food, Drug, and Cosmetics Act, anything that affects the structure of the body, as fat melting creams promise to do, are classified as drugs.

BUT DOES IT *Work?*

Enough of this alarmist babble! Do the creams work? Will they shrink your thighs down by two inches an hour? Who cares about the health risks! Breathing is a health risk! Do the creams work?

Unfortunately, not many studies have been done. The few that have been done, however, have not supported the claims made by all these late night infomercials, magazine ads, or Web sites. Dr. Leroy Young of Washington University conducted a study of fat melting creams and found that 16 out of 17 women found no improvement in their thighs after an eight-week trial. More studies need to be done, investigating the dangers and results, but thus far evidence suggests these creams can't keep the advertisers' promise of effectively melting your fat away into thin air.

Are you really that surprised? And who is that one out of 17 it did work for?

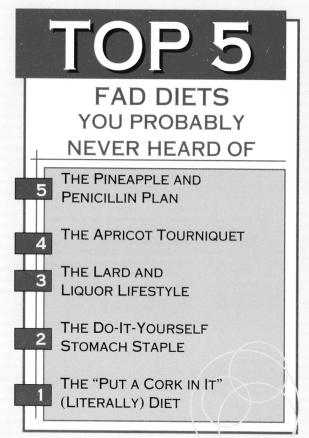

FAD DIETS, OR: WHAT'VE YOU GOT TO LOSE?

In the beginning of the Famous-Name Diet Plan Universe, there was Weight Watchers. And Weight Watchers begat Jenny Craig. And Jenny Craig begat Slim-Fast. And Slim-Fast begat Nutri-System. And Nutri-System begat Richard Simmons's Deal-A-Meal. These diet plans became so amazingly successful, that every putz with a vision of how to combine celery and cottage cheese asked himself, "Hey, why can't I begat my own diet plan, make a fortune, and quit my job taking photos at the DMV?"

Apparently, this is exactly what has happened. What follows are some little-known diet fads to compare with the latest "milk of yak/organic Vidalia onion" craze.

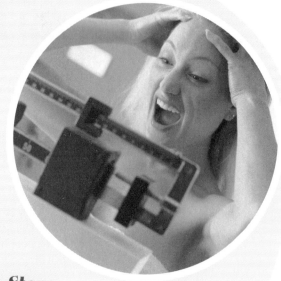

The Stone Age Diet

You must grow or kill everything you eat, and wear leopard skins while you do so. After as little as three months, you become an expert on soil conditions and outrunning livestock. Cave drawings of Twinkies and Milk Duds are strictly forbidden.

TOP 5 FAD DIETS YOU PROBABLY NEVER HEARD OF

5 THE PINEAPPLE AND PENICILLIN PLAN

4 THE APRICOT TOURNIQUET

3 THE LARD AND LIQUOR LIFESTYLE

2 THE DO-IT-YOURSELF STOMACH STAPLE

1 THE "PUT A CORK IN IT" (LITERALLY) DIET

The Yoga Diet

While seated in the Lotus Position, you repeat your healthy food word mantra, such as "carrot," over and over and over again, for hours on end, focusing on the mental image of a carrot. By the end of the day, you have leg cramps, and are so bored, angry, and frustrated, you lose your appetite.

The John McEnroe Diet

Halfway through your supermarket shopping spree, you get into a no-holds-barred shouting match with the store manager. He has you thrown out, without your groceries. 'Nuff said.

The Exxon Valdez Diet

You get drunk and spill tons of oil all over your food, rendering it inedible. You enlist the aid of volunteers to help you salvage what you can, which turns out coincidentally to add up to your allowable daily calorie count, anyway.

The Iraqi Diet

If you cheat, you have to cut off your hands.

The Amish Diet

You can eat anything you want, but you have to buggy-race to the store to get it, raise a barn after you eat it, and then hammer a hex sign over your home if you cheated.

The David Letterman Diet

Before you eat anything, you need to make up a funny top-ten list of the reasons why you should be allowed to eat it. Then, each bite you take must be preceded by a Stupid Food Trick.

The Woodstock Diet

All food must be consumed in the nude, during a rainstorm, while covered in mud. Don't eat the brown food. They are currently looking for a new spokesperson to replace David Crosby, who was never able to recover emotionally from the charge that he looks like he ate Stills and Nash.

The Los Angeles Diet

People who live outside Los Angeles are bussed in and forced to breathe the air and observe the crime, poverty, pollution, and quest for fame and fortune at any price. At that point, if they have any appetite left, they may eat what they want.

The Yoko Ono Diet

While eating, you must listen to her music. The higher the fat content, the louder the music must be played. This is the most successful diet of the last ten years. Top fashion models swear by it. Even Marlon Brando is giving it serious consideration.

The Haiti Diet

A voodoo curse is placed upon you. If you eat anything forbidden, you spend the rest of your life with a chicken's head replacing your own.

The *Baywatch* Diet

Arrangements are made that in exactly two months from the present, you will be appearing on an episode of *Baywatch*, wearing either a thong bikini for women, or a tiny Speedo swimsuit for men. Talk about having motivation.

The John Wayne Bobbitt Diet

You can eat anything you want, but your loved one must prepare it for you, at your bedside, with a huge carving knife, while you sleep. When you wake up, invariably, you get a big surprise. Also known as the Trust Diet.

The Amtrak Diet

You're on the train and attempt to eat as much as you can before the next train crash. Average meal time is thirteen minutes, so there are very few overweight folks on this diet plan.

The Nancy Kerrigan Diet

Each time you go over your caloric or fat limit, some goon comes out and whacks you in the knee. You cry out, "Why? Why me?" A booming voice responds, "Because you cheated on your diet!" You mutter, under your breath, "This is so corny."

The Carlos the Jackal Diet

You're allowed to eat virtually anything you please, but each dessert or high-fat item must be consumed on a different continent, under an assumed name. Those on this diet who recognize one another are allowed to acknowledge each other only with the code phrase "The pork chop fries at midnight."

The Anna Nicole Smith Diet

You are trained to develop a taste for 89-year old shoe leather. Yes, it's disgusting, but sometimes you have to sacrifice for a few years to attain your goal. But if anyone asks, you really do love the shoe leather. Honest. No, really.

The LaToya Jackson Diet

No food. You just stand around and criticize the other diets.

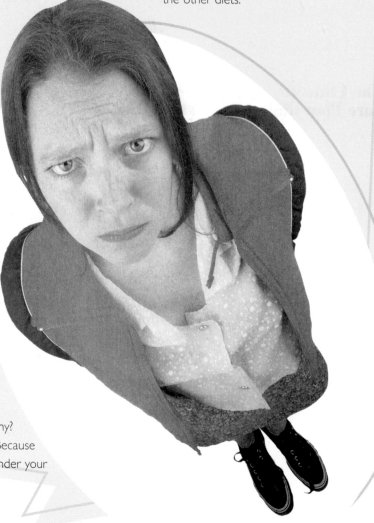

The Ted Kennedy Diet

You have to chase down your food in your underwear.

The Post Office Diet

Anything is allowed, but you have to eat it so slowly that you annoy everyone around you.

The Hard Copy Diet

You are only allowed to have food in your mouth while some shameful secret of your past is being revealed.

The Clinton Health Care Plan Diet

You may eat anything you like, you're just unable to pass it.

The Heidi Fleiss Diet

You end up looking great, because you yourself don't eat; you just gather the freshest, most attractive food in town, and rent it out for big bucks to the major eaters.

The Roseanne Diet

A big favorite. If you're caught cheating, you simply blame it on one of your 27 personalities.

The Shirley MacLaine Diet

Another "binge blamer." If you fall off the weight wagon, simply blame it on some fatso in a former life.

DIET DIARY 1: DOESN'T SHOPPING FOR DIET PILLS BURN CALORIES?

Of course, the United States' multibillion-dollar diet industry is betting on the fact that thin will be in a whole lot longer, as in, forever. For while Fen-Phen and its victims may have come and gone, there are still millionaires who made enough money off of both to happily retire because of its brief stint as the dietetic flavor of the month.

ANOREXIA SPLURGOSA

"That's it," you finally decided after yet another weekend of dining out, dining in, and dining in between and then trying to slip into yet another pair of business slacks that don't quite fit anymore for work on Monday morning. "It is time to go on a diet. Once and for all. Period. End of story."

Of course, this isn't the first time you've made the "diet decision." Your garage is filled with dusty diet books and exercise equipment, mute witnesses to your fitness flights of fancy over the years, which now stand sentinel, waiting for new victims to join their ranks when your latest "fitness fad" is over and done with, as it inevitably will be.

You decide, however, that you are done with all of that. No more books written by chubby doctors or aging sports stars. No more tummy tuckers or thigh tighteners hawked by fading starlets or sitcom survivors on late night infomercials.

You are in search of the sure thing. The no-fail. The guarantee. And so, armed with a will to lose weight without having to actually change or modify your behavior, you head for the local pharmacy and scour the "dietary aids" section for a quick cure-all.

And so you stock up on the pills, the gums, the dietetic chocolate cubes, the shakes, and the bars. After all, they sell it in the stores. They're "doctor recommended." They must work. Why didn't you think of this before?

Of course, you *have* thought of this before. You've even actually *done* all of this before. And, of course, it failed miserably. However, that was before the diet revolution and all of the new products out on the market. Certainly they've improved on all of that stuff by now. Right?

Unfortunately, as you soon find out, nothing much has changed at all. The pills make you high and, as soon as you stop going to the bathroom 22 times a day and your hands stop shaking, you crave more food than ever! The chocolate squares just make you want the real thing. The shakes—ditto. The bars, even more so.

By the end of the week, you've gained three pounds and have spent as much money in the vending machine at work as you did on your initial investment of dietary supplements.

As you bag said supplements up and stow them in the garage garbage can, you glance for a minute at the rest of your fitness fad failures and wonder if it might not be time to dust a few off and start anew, the old fashioned way, with blood, sweat, and carrot sticks.

"Nah," you think as you reach for the TV remote. "In a few hours some of those nifty infomercials will be on and I can get some new ideas. Until then, I'll just sit here with my credit card ready and polish off the rest of those chocolate squares, diet shakes, and energy bars I 'forgot' to throw away."

DIET DIARY II:
SEARCHING FOR
MR. ENERGY BAR

In my 24 years of life, I have tried just about every diet known to man. No, seriously, I have searched high and low for every diet possibility and found a world of chaos, contradictions, and confusion. Every diet tells you it is the best. Every diet tells you fast weight loss is ahead. Some even warn you against losing too *much* weight! From my own experience, I can tell you that finding the diet that is right for you is a perilous journey, so fasten your girdle and let's begin.

Let's start at the top of the food chain, the government recommended diet, you know, that little pyramid thing. Protein and dairy at the top in the smallest portions and veggies, fruit, and bread at the bottom. I wholeheartedly disagree with this diet! If I eat as much bread

as they recommend, my stomach will feel like I swallowed a rock. I gained three pounds in one week following these guidelines. In my opinion, that cannot be considered success.

Next in line, those prepackaged food diet centers. I won't name names, but we all know who they are. These places bring you into their office, where you sit down with an attractive skinny person, who explains to you why you can't lose weight without them and tries to convince you to join their program for only $9 plus the cost of food. Sounds pretty good right? Menus planned out for you, no measuring, perfect portions, no shopping, what could be better? Well, the food for one! Tiny, tasteless portions are the typical fare for these places, combined with an exorbitant price. Kinda makes you wonder what you are really paying for—I'd say that attractive skinny woman's salary.

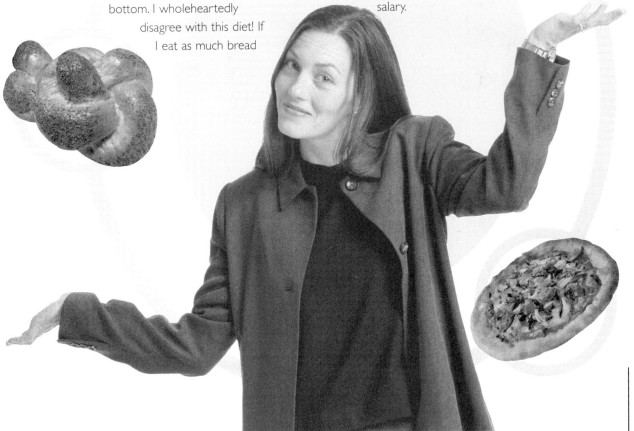

Moving on, we'll hit the world of diet pills, starting with the latest fad. These pills promote themselves as "fat busters" attaching themselves to fat so it cannot be absorbed into the system. Where does it go then, you may ask? Believe me, you will find out about six hours later. Side effects of these pills, packed with chitosan, are loose, oily bowel movements. Loose, oily bowel movements? More like explosions of matter that no human body should have to endure. Unless you can always be within running distance of a toilet, steer clear!

And just to let you know, a pill cannot speed up your metabolism, no matter what they tell you. They can speed up your heartbeat, they can speed up your brain, mostly because their active ingredients are a form of speed, whether chemical or herbal. If this is your thing, more power to ya, but I tend to not enjoy my heart pounding, teeth chattering, and thoughts swirling around in my head like a tornado. Pass!

How about all those crazy, weird food diets? There's the all you can eat cabbage soup diet. Doesn't that sound appealing? Tastes like a cooked sneaker and gives you the runs—not good. How about Day 1 eat all the fruit you want, Day 2 eat all the veggies you want, Day 3 drink only fruit juice, Days 5-7 eat veggie soup? This diet just confused my poor little belly, and I gained 2 pounds—also not good. How about the no dairy, no sugar diet? Hmm let's see, weak bones and no ice cream? I don't think so.

I've read every diet book I could get my hands on and every diet contradicts the next. It just sounds like they're making it up. So I decided to take my weight in my own hands and devise my own diets. Okay, we'll start with the grapefruit and grape nuts diet. You've heard the rumors about grapefruits, cutting through the fat in your body? Well, I figured grape nuts had the same beginning so, why not? Why not? Because after a few days, the grapefruit had caused sores in my mouth that the grape nuts irritated. Scratch that diet.

How about white rice and veggies? No fat in that, right? I ate rice and veggies for a whole month, nothing else. By the end of the month I had gained 15 pounds. 15 pounds! I didn't even cheat! I did better eating whatever I wanted, at least I was maintaining that way, not gaining!

Finally, at the end of my rope, I found a diet that worked for me. Really, I did! It was one of those high protein-low carb diets they warn you not to go on. This was the one diet that I could stick to, had lots of food options, and ice cream every night! All the meat, cheese, and green veggies I can eat during the day and a bowl of ice cream every night! I lost 70 pounds in four months. (Okay, give or take 69 pounds.)

True, there is a chance your cholesterol may go up, they say heart disease is down the road—but I think I'd rather be thin now and worry about that later. Now, this diet isn't for everyone. I put a friend on this and she gained three pounds in the first three days. Usually, a history of alcoholism and diabetes in your family will be most conducive to this diet. Of course, once you stop eating this way the weight starts to come back, I know from personal experience.

Basically, all I can tell you is that you need to find what's right for you, what fits your lifestyle, and what you can live with. You'll have to be on it for the rest of your life, so choose wisely. Personally, I think I'm gonna stick to that corny elementary school joke diet: the seafood diet. I see food, I eat it.

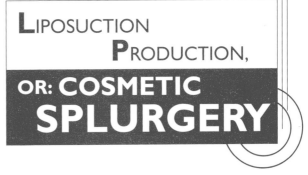

LIPOSUCTION PRODUCTION, OR: COSMETIC SPLURGERY

Plug a vacuum into a straw and combine it with a certified, licensed physician and you don't just get a new cosmetic surgery procedure, you get a national obsession that does for thighs and hips what Dow and Corning did for breasts, only, in the opposite direction. Don't believe it? Why not consider this little thigh tale.

THIGH MASTER

You remember it quite clearly. That day you saw your first-ever liposuction procedure in televised bits and snippets on *Oprah*. The sucking sounds in the background of the hidden camera video, the violent stabbing of the lengthy straw and vacuum contraption and the receptacle at the doctor's protectively bootied feet slowly filling with human cottage cheese in a delightfully realistic shade of nicotine yellow.

Of course, Oprah had meant the broadcast as a cautionary tale, frequently quoting alarming statistics about such cosmetic surgical procedures in between graphic videotape from the clandestine footage of an actual operation. Still, you just concentrated on the "After" pictures. Which, when the swelling had finally gone down and the patient was able to get up and walk on her own two feet after a brief two months, were not exactly extraordinary, but still beat the 8 months of Stairmasters it would have taken for you to attain the same results. Since then, of course, you've conducted further research on your own. Magazine articles,

medical Web pages, anonymous phone calls to plastic surgeons with a pseudo-disguised voice, etc. A file folder in between the grocery coupons and hair dryer warrantees holds the various clippings, printouts, brochures, and price lists you've managed to amass in a few brief months of extensive research.

Finally, you decide to take the plunge and actually consult a licensed physician, in his office, *sans* disguise or fake voice boxes. You consult your "fat" file of

information one last time, choose the most local practitioner available, call his secretary, and make an appointment.

Relieved, you write down a date and time mere weeks in the future, circle it on your calendar, and proceed to retire your walking shoes for the duration, confident in the fact that your thighs will soon be firm, young, and supple again. Just like they were when you were eighteen, okay, twenty years old—*without* the lacing up at 7 in the morning before work, or, worse, traipsing around your office building parking lot six arduous times during your lunch break in the always fashionable power suit and tennis shoes combo.

You begin indulging in late-night snacks, a novelty for you. Vienna Fingers and Malomars and a different flavor of International coffee each night after work.

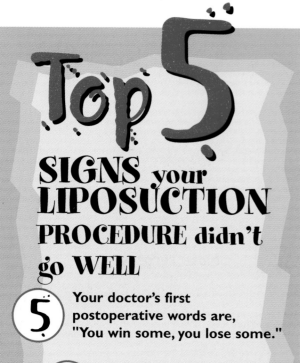

Top 5

SIGNS your LIPOSUCTION PROCEDURE didn't go WELL

5 Your doctor's first postoperative words are, "You win some, you lose some."

4 Your friends keep asking when you're going to have it done.

3 *60 Minutes* asks for permission to televise it on an episode titled, "Quacks."

2 Your boyfriend's sudden fondness for the word "botched."

1 Your doctor calls to ask if that "big ass, plastic straw" he left in your thigh is causing any discomfort.

Of course, your work slacks begin to grow a little snug in the intervening weeks, but you're quite sure this will all be taken care of in one simple, hours-long, extremely painful, not to mention unnatural, surgical procedure that is now less than one week away from becoming a reality.

So you switch to skirts for the time being and continue your midnight snack routine. Until, one late night, too hyped up to sleep from a bad combination of caramel, chocolate, and nougat, you are flipping through the channels and come across one of those hard-hitting, exposé/documentary type films HBO likes to toss on every once in a while in between *Inside the NFL* and the after-dark skinflicks.

Of course, it's about strippers and their not so charmed life, but while you're up, you set aside the clicker and indulge yourself. Eventually, a young woman named "Double-D Desire" decides, in a gut-wrenching cinematic moment, to undergo a breast reduction.

Her quack of a cinematic doctor, however, seeing dollar signs and an autographed picture for his waiting room, persuades the impressionable nineteen year old to undergo liposuction while she's under the knife, despite the fact that you could bounce quarters off of her cellulite-free thighs and dimes off of her perfect rear-end.

Since the strip club (whose owner Desire just happens to be dating) is paying for the surgical procedure, she giggles and nods and is soon splayed out on a surgical table, unconscious, her skin the color of a dead fish's belly, drool running down her cheeks as the camera focuses in on a hairy but gloved hand as it grips the end of a long, thin vacuum tube mercilessly while ramming it into Debra's thighs as if he were sanding an oak table that needed refinishing.

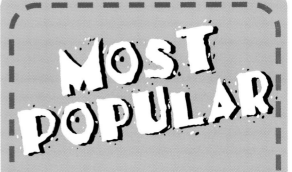

Cosmetic SURGERIES

- Breast enlargement
- Breast reduction
- Breast lift
- Liposuction
- Facelift
- Nose surgery
- Hair removal surgery
- Laser skin resurfacing
- Lip implants
- Laser eye surgery
- Teeth bleaching
- Tattoo removal
- Tummy tuck
- Forehead lift
- Eyelid surgery
- Hair replacement

Obviously, Oprah had settled on a tamer version of the procedure for her episode, perhaps due to the fact that the bootlegged butchery you are currently witnessing might have given her show an NC-17 rating for the afternoon. Reddish, pinkish, yellowish goo fills the doctor's industrial strength straw, its flatulent flow disrupted only intermittently by huge chunks of fat that clog it with a sound worthy of The *Exorcist* sound track.

The outline of the sinister straw pokes, prods, and peels the poor girl's thighs for what seems like hours, until finally they show her being wheeled in a morphine induced coma to her boyfriend's pick-up truck where, despite massive amounts of medication, she screams in pain at being placed on the front seat.

Quickly dialing your doctor's answering service, despite the late hour, you leave a vague message about having to leave the country unexpectedly for tax evasion purposes, and then hang up the phone quickly. Emptying the fridge of your sweet tooth shenanigans, you bring the dusty tennis shoes out of your closet and lay them next to tomorrow's power suit, wondering if the ladies in the "Lunchtime Walking Club" will let you back in after dumping them unceremoniously after your first doctor's appointment weeks earlier.

It is not an entirely uncommon sight these days to witness fellow shoppers staring intently at an array of prepackaged food, just before they suddenly recoil in horror and stomp the offending package as if it were an unsightly cockroach in their closet back home. This involuntary action is then quickly followed by a look of disgust and incomprehensible muttering as the shopper abruptly sweeps past the hordes of unsuspecting

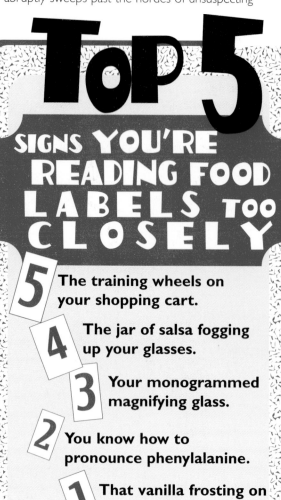

TOP 5
SIGNS YOU'RE READING FOOD LABELS TOO CLOSELY

5 The training wheels on your shopping cart.

4 The jar of salsa fogging up your glasses.

3 Your monogrammed magnifying glass.

2 You know how to pronounce phenylalanine.

1 That vanilla frosting on your nose.

cracker connoisseurs and waddles over to the ice cream freezer for a cart full of Klondike bars and Fudgsicles.

Who can blame them? After all, this is the era of nutrition labels. Nutrition labels that have scammed their way into the world of the American consumer. But wait, there's more. This craze does not discriminate. We are talking about an equal opportunity obsession here.

Perhaps older, wiser individuals would not be taken in by this phenomena. But an encounter at the local food store will wean a person off that assumption with quickness. Unfortunately, youths have succumbed to this tri-focal trend as well. Sadly, even the beacons of hope that we call the country's future leaders have been fooled by this sorry display of propaganda.

Ask the average college student about the downfalls of unsaturated fat intake and you'll get a blank stare. But ask the same person why they read labels and they'll give you a well rehearsed, "I'm watching my fat intake." Yeah, okay. Weren't you just proudly discussing your latest drinking feat to some avid listeners, who can only dream of one day following in your illustrious shoes? Health conscious are we? Sure. And the guys at the local pizza place don't happen to know that the "#5 with extra toppings" is your calling card.

It used to be that everyone was just worried about too much red meat in their diets. Now all of a sudden everyone has become a self-proclaimed dietitian. It has become acceptable to inspect various food packages in order to read that tiny

TRICEPS *tip*

When reading food labels, take your time. Avoid rushing into a purchase just because something says "1 calorie per serving" on the front label. Turning the product over and reading more closely, you might just find that the package contains 78 servings!

snippet of information the FDA has deemed infallible. Low fat, Reduced fat, Less fat, Non-fat—what exactly is going on here? So, with the influx of information, are Americans suddenly becoming healthier and more fit than ever before? Judging by the latest statistics put out by the American Medical Association and the rise in obesity, not quite.

Maybe there is no answer. Maybe Americans are trapped, forced to go to their local food stores and mindlessly hold up every item and announce the numbers on the side of each item in their shopping carts to no one in particular. People have been sentenced to a life of label reading with no working knowledge of what exactly it is they're looking for. It is one huge conspiracy. We will never know when the madness will end.

So do yourself a favor: Next time you find yourself browsing through the aisles of your local market and you happen upon one of these "label pushers," don't panic. Just smile and continue on your way. And don't forget to pick up some ice cream on your way out.

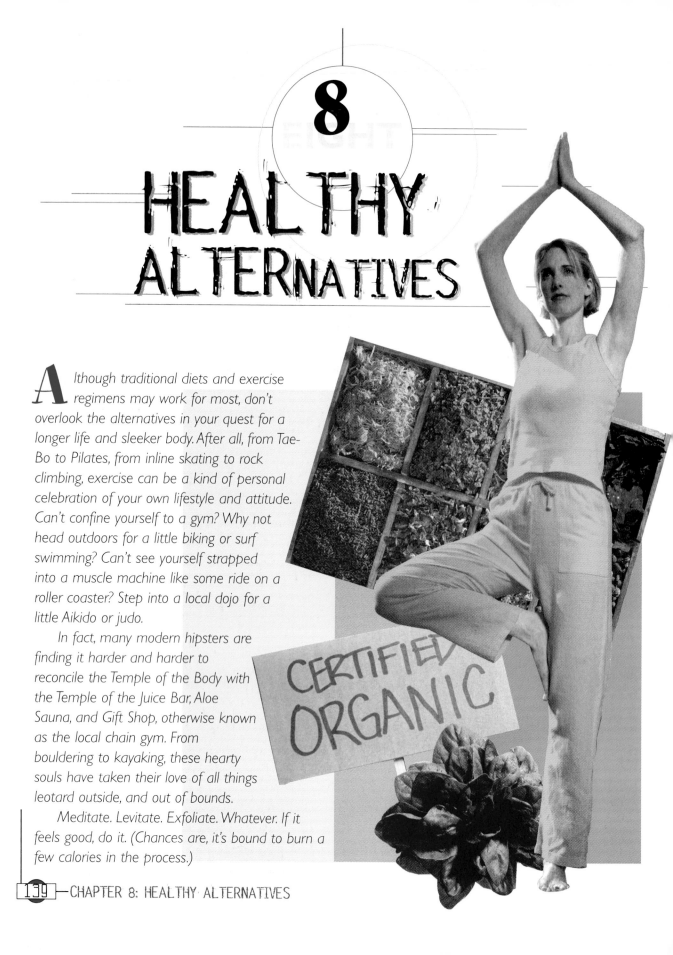

8

HEALTHY ALTERNATIVES

Although traditional diets and exercise regimens may work for most, don't overlook the alternatives in your quest for a longer life and sleeker body. After all, from Tae-Bo to Pilates, from inline skating to rock climbing, exercise can be a kind of personal celebration of your own lifestyle and attitude. Can't confine yourself to a gym? Why not head outdoors for a little biking or surf swimming? Can't see yourself strapped into a muscle machine like some ride on a roller coaster? Step into a local dojo for a little Aikido or judo.

In fact, many modern hipsters are finding it harder and harder to reconcile the Temple of the Body with the Temple of the Juice Bar, Aloe Sauna, and Gift Shop, otherwise known as the local chain gym. From bouldering to kayaking, these hearty souls have taken their love of all things leotard outside, and out of bounds.

Meditate. Levitate. Exfoliate. Whatever. If it feels good, do it. (Chances are, it's bound to burn a few calories in the process.)

CERTIFIED ORGANIC

YOU GO, YO GA! OR: (HUMAN) PRETZELS ANYONE?

Consider this your lucky day. We're going to let you in on something that can ease stress, heal old injuries, protect you from new ones, burn lots of calories, and demand less than two hours a week. No, it's not that. (We said two hours, not two minutes, stud boy.)

Like the chicken soup stock in your great-grandmother's freezer, yoga has been around for centuries. We all suspect that yoga is probably good for us, but we're no doubt put off by our belief that there's some mystical, Eastern aura to it, that it's taught by long-bearded swamis with unpronounceable 17-syllable names, and that it involves twisting our bodies into configurations seen primarily in the video section of Lou's Hot & Nasty Hardcore EmPORNium.

While all this is true, yoga nonetheless has a strong U.S. following—six million limber souls, according to the latest Roper poll. One school of yoga is called power yoga. It is drawn from a branch of classic yoga called ashtanga, which, loosely translated, means, "Oh, dear Vishnu, that really hurts!" In a typical power yoga session, there are no pauses between the poses. It's just one continuous, heart-pounding, heavy-breathing, sweat-inducing session—kind of like prom night, but without all the heaving from consuming apricot brandy and Cheetos.

OUCH!

There are a number of intriguing principles behind power yoga. One is that some exercises can hurt as much as they help. That is, you can be strong from lifting weights, or aerobically fit from running, but still be tight and injury-prone because of the one-dimensionality of your workouts. (This also illustrates one of the foremost tenets of yoga—belittling all other forms of exercise.)

TRICEPS tip

Avoid caffeine or overdoing any beverage before your yoga class. Concentration in this healthful endeavor is key, and an overactive or full bladder isn't going to help you tap into your inner you if you're "meditating" on when you can take your next bathroom break.

Another principle is that stretching (i.e., two or three quick stretches before a yoga workout) is a waste of time, since muscles must be warm to be malleable, and generating this healing heat is what yoga is all about.

Still skeptical? Practitioners of power yoga include Kareem Abdul-Jabbar, Sting, and the men's varsity swim team at Columbia University—all of whom will be appearing together in the new, yoga-themed, NBC sitcom, *Who's the Swami?* (Just kidding.)

Ready to give it a try? Hey, come back here! At least listen to these hints for a more productive workout.

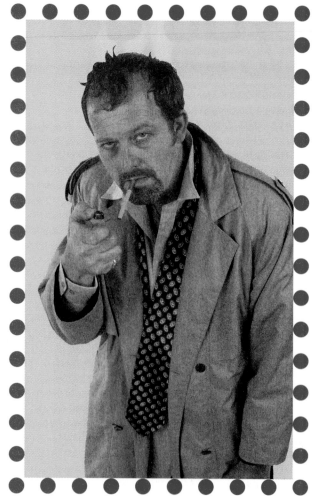

TOP 5

SIGNS YOU'RE NOT "INTO" YOUR YOGA CLASS

5 "Excuse me, miss, this is a no-smoking dojo."

4 Your inflatable girlfriend/workout mat.

3 "Barkeep, another double for me and Ms. Fonda."

2 You're munching pretzels, not bending like one.

1 "Yeah, listen Swami. When does that guy from Tae-Bo get here?"

Your exercise clothing should allow for complete freedom of movement. If you wear pants, they should be loose enough for a sheep to fit in them with you. Keep your attention fixed on what you are doing. Poise and balance should be maintained at all times.

Do the recommended exercises at least three days a week. Set aside 15 minutes for the opening week's exercises and 30 minutes for the closing week's workouts.

Remember that deep relaxation is a duet of the body and mind in repose.

For better balance, concentrate on your breathing and gaze out at some fixed point, such as the neighborhood children looking into your window and giggling.

Don't get discouraged. Much like applying for unemployment, it may take two to four weeks to start realizing benefits.

YOGA POSTURES

Fundamental yoga positions for the beginner to use to start his or her future life as a contortionist are simple. They require almost no equipment, except perhaps for a comfortable mat or rug and the appropriately funky attire. And they can be performed in any order. Start slowly and listen to your body, and enjoy your yoga experience.

Sitting/Easy Position

This is a starting position that helps focus awareness on breathing and the body. It also helps strengthen the lower back, the groin, and hips. Begin by sitting cross-legged, with your hands on your knees. Sit still, and focus on your breathing. Keep your spine straight and push your buttocks toward the floor. At the same time, allow your knees to gently lower as well. Still in this sitting position, take five to ten slow, deep breaths. On the final inhale, raise your arms slowly over your head. Next, exhale and bring your arms down slowly, repeating this process five to seven times. From here, you should be ready to move on to a more challenging position.

Dog and Cat

This intermediate position serves to increase the flexibility of your spine. Once you've been in this position for a minute or two, you'll realize the origins of its name. Begin the dog portion of this two-pronged position by kneeling

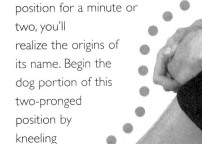

on your hands and knees. Remember to keep your hands just in front of your shoulders and your legs only about hip-width apart. As you inhale, tilt your tailbone and pelvis up, while letting your spine downward, at the same time lifting your head up. (Unless you're a porn star, this action may take some getting used to, so practice first.)

Remember, as is the case with all of these positions, move slowly and stretch gently. As you exhale, move into the cat position by reversing the spinal bend, tilting the pelvis down, drawing the spine up and pulling the chest and stomach in. Repeat several times, flowing (big yoga word) smoothly from dog into cat and back again.

Mountain

This position, like so many in yoga, serves to improve not only your posture, but your balance and your self-awareness as well.

Begin this position by standing with your feet together, your hands at your sides, and your eyes looking straight ahead. Raise your toes and fan them open before placing them back down on the floor so that your heel, the outside of your foot, your toes, and the ball of your foot are all in contact with the floor. Next, tilt your pubic bone slightly forward and raise your chest up and out. Raise your head as well, and lengthen your neck by lifting the base of your skull toward the ceiling. Stretch the pinky on each hand downward, then balance that movement by stretching your index fingers. Breathe. Hold the posture, but try not to tense up. Breathe again. As you inhale, imagine the breath coming up through the floor, rising through your legs, then your torso, and on up into your head. Reverse the process on the exhale and watch your breath as it passes down from your head, through your chest and stomach, legs, and feet. On your next inhale, raise your arms over your head and hold for several breaths. Lower your arms on an exhale.

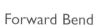

Forward Bend

Despite its lack of a mystical, or even comical, name, this basic position stretches the legs and spine, rests the heart and neck, and relaxes the mind and body. So what's not to like?

Begin by standing straight up in a pose such as Mountain. Inhale and raise your arms overhead. Exhale, then bend at the hips while bringing your arms forward and down until you touch the floor. (Don't worry about bending your knees, especially if you're feeling stiff.) Grasp your ankles (in prison, this is called "assuming the position") and breathe several times. Repeat this position three to five times. On your last bend, hold the position for five to ten breaths.

The Triangle

This familiar pose from your junior high school PE classes stretches the spine, opens the torso, and improves your balance as well as your concentration. Start with your legs spread several feet apart, but comfortably, and your feet parallel. Turn your left foot 90 degrees to the left and your right foot about 45 degrees inward. Inhale and raise both arms so that they are parallel with the floor. Exhale, then turn your head to the left and look down your left arm toward your outstretched fingers.

Take a deep breath and stretch outward to the left, tilting the left hip down and the right hip up. When you've stretched as far as you can, bend at the waist, letting your left hand reach down and come to rest against the inside of your calf, while your right arm points straight up. Turn and look up at your right hand. Breathe deeply for several breaths. Inhale, then straighten up. Exhale, then lower your arms. Put your hands on your hips and pivot on your heels, bringing your feet to face front. Repeat the posture on the other side.

Warrior

This fierce sounding but simple position strengthens your legs and arms and improves balance and concentration. Begin, yet again, in the Mountain pose with your feet together and your hands by your sides. Slide your feet several feet apart. Turn your right foot about 45 degrees to the left and your left foot about 90 degrees to the left so that it is pointing straight out to the side. Slowly bend the left knee until your thigh is parallel with the floor. Gently raise your arms over your head as you breathe. Next, slowly lower them until your left arm is pointing straight ahead and your right arm is pointing back. Concentrate on a spot in front of you and breathe carefully. Take four or five deep breaths, then lower your arms and bring your legs together before reversing the position.

The Cobra

Another fierce-sounding position that is deceptively simple, this position stretches the spine and strengthens your back and arms. Begin by laying down on your stomach. Be careful to keep your legs together, with your arms at your sides and close to your body, with your hands by your chest, as if you were preparing to do push-ups. As you inhale carefully, slowly raise your head and chest as high as it will go. Keep your head up and your chest out. Breathe several times and then come down again. Repeat as necessary. When you've gone as high as you can, gently raise yourself on your arms, stretching your spine even more. Only go as far as you are comfortable. Your pelvis should always remain on the floor. Breathe several times before coming down. Repeat as desired.

Downward Facing Dog

Not only does it have one of the coolest names in yoga, but this position also builds strength, flexibility, and awareness. It even stretches the spine and hamstrings and rests the heart, especially if you've been doing a few of the more strenuous positions from above! Start on your hands and knees, as in Dog and Cat, and keep your legs about hip width apart and your arms shoulder width apart. Your middle fingers should be parallel, pointing straight ahead. Inhale and curl your toes under, as if getting ready to stand on your toes. Exhale and straighten your legs, while pushing upward with your arms. The goal is to lengthen the spine while keeping your legs straight and your feet flat on the ground—although it's okay to bend the knees at first. Hold the position for a few breaths. Come down and exhale. Repeat several times, synchronizing with your breath: up on the exhale and down on the inhale.

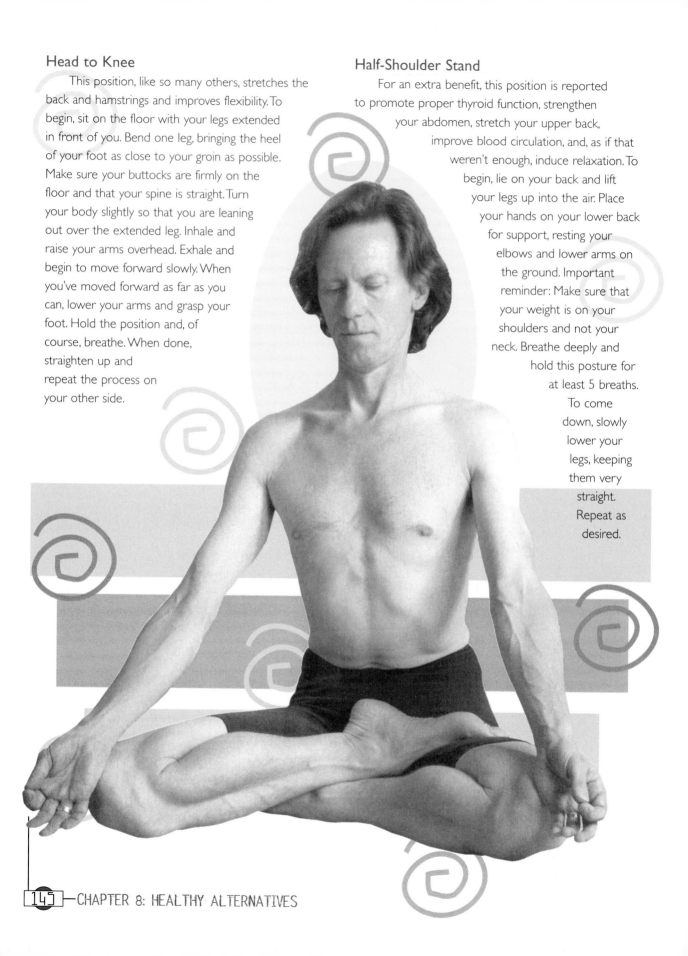

Head to Knee

This position, like so many others, stretches the back and hamstrings and improves flexibility. To begin, sit on the floor with your legs extended in front of you. Bend one leg, bringing the heel of your foot as close to your groin as possible. Make sure your buttocks are firmly on the floor and that your spine is straight. Turn your body slightly so that you are leaning out over the extended leg. Inhale and raise your arms overhead. Exhale and begin to move forward slowly. When you've moved forward as far as you can, lower your arms and grasp your foot. Hold the position and, of course, breathe. When done, straighten up and repeat the process on your other side.

Half-Shoulder Stand

For an extra benefit, this position is reported to promote proper thyroid function, strengthen your abdomen, stretch your upper back, improve blood circulation, and, as if that weren't enough, induce relaxation. To begin, lie on your back and lift your legs up into the air. Place your hands on your lower back for support, resting your elbows and lower arms on the ground. Important reminder: Make sure that your weight is on your shoulders and not your neck. Breathe deeply and hold this posture for at least 5 breaths. To come down, slowly lower your legs, keeping them very straight. Repeat as desired.

The Bridge

This relaxing position increases flexibility and suppleness, strengthens the lower back and abdominal muscles, and clears the chest. To begin, lie on your back with your knees up and your hands at your side. Your feet should be near your buttocks and about six inches apart. Next, gently raise and lower your butt. Then, slowly, raise the tailbone and continue lifting until your entire back is arched upward. Push firmly with your feet, while keeping your knees straight and close together. Breathe deeply into your chest. Clasp your hands under your back and push against the floor. Take five slow, deep breaths before coming down slowly and repeating.

The Corpse

An appropriate way to end your yoga session, this deceptively simple position relaxes and refreshes the body and mind, relieves stress and anxiety, and supposedly quiets the mind (hence the name). Possibly the most important posture, the Corpse is usually performed at the end of a session, the goal being conscious relaxation. Begin by lying on your back, with your feet slightly apart and your arms at your sides with the palms facing up. Close your eyes and take several slow, deep breaths as you allow your body to sink to the ground. Then simply breathe and relax as you stay in the pose for at least five to 10 minutes. See why it's called the Corpse?

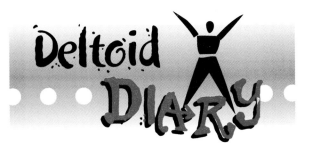

Deltoid DIARY

Fitness Guru Gripe

I don't know about you, but I am getting really sick of everyone making a big deal out of the "health craze." If I go to the gym five times a week, I work out too much. If I eat a salad for dinner, I must be on a diet. If I avoid the chips while watching Monday night football, I'm calorie counting. Since when did it become such an unusual thing to be—dare I say—healthy?

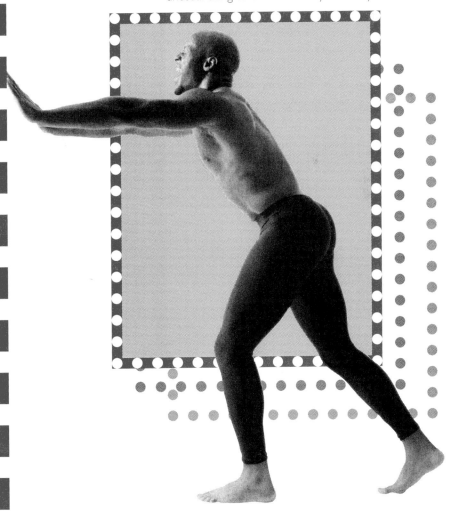

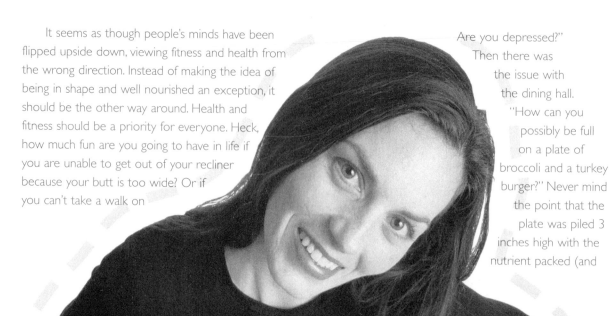

It seems as though people's minds have been flipped upside down, viewing fitness and health from the wrong direction. Instead of making the idea of being in shape and well nourished an exception, it should be the other way around. Health and fitness should be a priority for everyone. Heck, how much fun are you going to have in life if you are unable to get out of your recliner because your butt is too wide? Or if you can't take a walk on the beach without stopping to gasp for air? Although it is a wonderful thing, being healthy has gotten a bad rep. It is embraced fanatically by those in the health conscious segment, but outsiders feeling that zealous overkill tend to put it down.

When I was a freshman in college, I used to attend two aerobics classes a day. Because I had such a handle on my studies, I had a lot of free time in the evenings. While everyone else was watching television and vegging out, I decided to make the most of my time and get in shape. Now, you would think my friends would commend me on my dedication to a healthy life, or think it was great that I had such a drive to be fit. Wrong. Instead of a thumbs up, I received a rush of concern, "Are you sure you're not exercising too much?" Or, "Gee, you go to the gym a lot, huh? Are you depressed?" Then there was the issue with the dining hall. "How can you possibly be full on a plate of broccoli and a turkey burger?" Never mind the point that the plate was piled 3 inches high with the nutrient packed (and pungent) green stuff. I just don't see why having broccoli for dinner needs to be made into an issue. Or even commented on. And just to ease the minds of everyone out there who feels the same way, there is nothing wrong with having vegetables and boiled chicken for dinner. Just because I don't like to slather my food in gravy doesn't mean I have an eating disorder. So I *like* fresh vegetables, so I actually *like* the taste of my food without fatty sauces. So I *like* water instead of sugary sodas. Sue me.

Being healthy is a good thing and it's unfair to make those who are conscious of their health and bodies feel like some sort of outcast or superhero. (Remember, Superman didn't have a lot of pals.) So enough with the looks toward that girl who is running past you, and enough with the snickering behind the back of the one who's in line at the salad bar. Instead, why not take that energy and take a hike. Now there's a concept.

VARICOSE VARIETY, OR: SPICING UP YOUR SWEAT LIFE

There are many ways to spice up your sweat life, and we're not talking about buying a new Kid Rock CD to listen to while strutting your stuff on the treadmill. If your workout has become as stale as the air in your gym locker, why not look to sports to spice things up?

Sure, it's been years since you played on a team, but you don't have to go to the Dodgers' spring training camp to add a curve ball to your workout routine. And don't rule out exercising with a partner, or even several. Studies have shown that working out with another like-minded soul motivates both of you, and often gets people out of the house when, if left to their own devices, they would have simply loafed on the couch for another couple of hours.

Furthermore, many organizations have sports teams that are always in need of a warm body. Softball, soccer, and volleyball are all physical activities that are not just good exercise, but great fun. Want more? Read along for a little example of how beneficial a little organized teamwork can be to your workout.

NET WORTH

If you asked a group of kids how much time they were spending at the "net," not one of them would think you were talking about tennis. What was chic in the '70s and '80s was abandoned for inline skating and golf in the early '90s. Participation in tennis may have dropped below that of dart throwing for a little while, but thanks to some grass roots efforts, tennis is set for a comeback.

Popularity in tennis vanished with the same vengeance as sideburns. Top professionals like John McEnroe and Chris Evert expressed embarrassment by the lack of interest in their sport. Courts everywhere were empty. Leagues dissolved. Interest in televising the big tournaments was minimal at best. Tennis was in trouble and people knew it. Tennis needed a Tiger Woods (or at least an Anna Kournikova . . . oh, wait). Tennis needed something sleek, magical, or sexy (or at least an Anna Kournikova . . . oh, wait). But first, tennis needed to get cheaper.

Clubs everywhere started offering free lessons. Kids became a target market, luring them away from other activities with free equipment and lessons. League play became less competitive and more fun. Now, once cracked courts that housed many varieties of weeds have been resurfaced and suddenly find themselves full once again.

There are good reasons for the return to this sport:

• Tennis is a lifelong sport. Almost anyone can learn to hit the ball over the net, and it is a sport people are proving you can play well into your nineties. How many sports can offer that?

• Tennis is a social sport. No matter what city you move to, if you play tennis, you'll have instant relationships. League play is also a great way to network.

• Tennis is good exercise. It has all the normal benefits of exercise, including lowering blood pressure, increasing heart rate, increasing muscle tone, and it is great for relieving aggression. Bad day at work? Smack

that ball! Husband left you with no gas? Smack! Husband just plain left you? Smack! Smack! Boss looked at his wristwatch when you walked into work two minutes late? Whack, whack, whack!

• Tennis is something you can do with your spouse or significant other. Whether you team up for doubles or face your better half from across the net, competitive fun is good for your relationship. Of course, acing your spouse every serve probably won't score you many affection points later.

• Tennis doesn't take an unreasonable amount of equipment. Rackets are made to last years. You don't need to wear anything fancy to enjoy the sport.

• Tennis puts you in the great outdoors. Get out in the air! Feel the sun on your shoulders.

• Tennis doesn't require all day to play. You don't need to reserve four hours to play one match. You don't need perfect conditions. Indoor courts offer an alternative activity in the frigid days of winter.

• Tennis is a relatively safe sport. In an age where people seem to want to scale cliffs, bungee jump off bridges, and ski down avalanche paths, isn't it refreshing to know you can still feel the thrill of sport without risking your life?

• Tennis is responsible for ... Anna Kournikova. Thank god for fuzzy green balls!

So, dust off that racket. It's probably under your eight-track tape player in the garage. Drag your buddy off the Internet. Buy a pack of strawberries and some skim milk (better for you than cream) and turn on just enough Wimbledon to get inspired. Then get out there and give your friend a little shot. As Groucho Marx said, "It's better to have lobbed and lost than never to have lobbed at all."

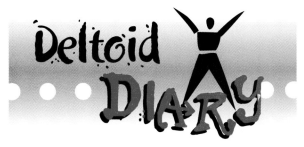

Recess for Grownups

I am eleven (or at least I was). Perhaps my greatest source of pride is that I am the second best girl at dodge ball in my class. I don't know if anyone else notices, but I know. I know how to throw the ball low and hard so that it hits the foot of someone on the other team before they can catch it. And I know how to not be afraid of the ball when it comes hurtling toward me, to get my hands and body around it so I can make a clean catch without it hitting me square in the face.

Sometimes we substitute soccer for dodge ball, but one day the boys decided not to let us play. We argued with one of the team captains, Ryan. The next day we were simply ignored. From that day on, the girls stood on the side and talked. Sports had become a dark place, and a place where I didn't go.

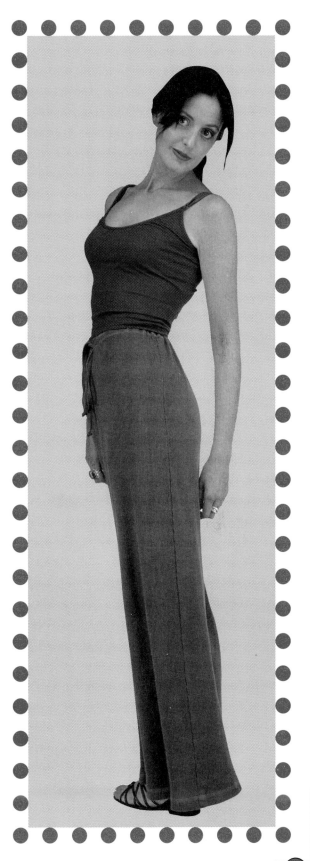

Fast forward. I am twenty-seven and becoming aware that my body is losing some of its tone. I panic. But, I calm down enough and come up with a plan. First, I start running. Then I join a gym and go to aerobics classes.

Then I begin to do ab workouts, weights, and soon I am admiring myself in the mirror, eager to get a boyfriend so I can show off my body even more. And I notice that I am getting sick less and that every time I exercise I am energized and happy. This is great. But I'm bored. Very bored. Although I always feel good after exercising, I consistently dread working out beforehand. I must drag myself to step class. I must throw myself into the pool to do laps. I must trick myself by taking a Discman and a magazine onto the treadmill, making believe it will be fun. But it's not. It's not fun at all.

Fast forward again. Now I'm twenty-nine. I have found a boyfriend to whom I can show off my body. He is English and wants to start a pick-up football game in the park. But since he is English, what he means is he wants to start a pick-up soccer game in the park. He convinces me to come along. I don't know what I'm doing. Wherever the ball is, that's where I run. When the ball is passed to me I kick out my foot to pass it back but it rolls clear under my leg and I feel ridiculous. When I do manage to kick it, it goes straight into the foot of someone from the opposing team. The ball comes at my head and I shield my face with my hands and hear everyone shout "handball!" at the top of their lungs. Naturally, the other team gets possession. I was supposed to hit it with my head. I think of Ryan on the playground. Then a tiny light breaks through. Despite this first, less than flawless performance, I show up every week. Two months later I am stopping the ball with my toes when it comes to me.

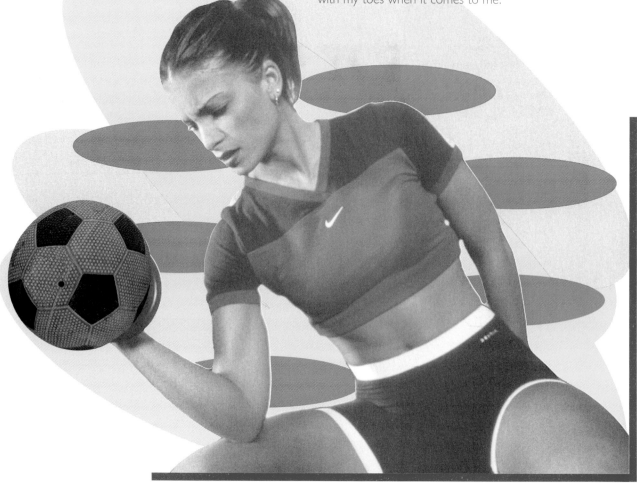

I am looking on the wings to see who to pass it to and then I do, angling it so no one opposing intercepts it. I myself wait on the wing, remaining open when we have possession, and when it comes lobbing through the air I butt it forward with my chest, then kick it ahead.

I watch the Spanish guy, Fernando, who is the best player. I watch how delicately he maneuvers the ball. I see that it is not a game of strength but of precision. All the American guys think they're playing football. The Spanish guy gently rolls it to me as the opposing goaltender blocks him from kicking it in the right corner. The left corner is wide open and I tap it forward and in—easy. I still have not hit the ball with my head.

Some months after I started playing soccer, my friend tells me that on Wednesday nights, a group of women play basketball. Wednesday night is step class but I decide to ditch it and go play hoops instead. I have some natural talents. I know to pass the ball low, under the reach of opposing players. I move constantly, getting and staying open. And I instinctively set a screen for my teammate as she goes in for the lay-up. If a gun were held to my head, though, I still couldn't sink a basket. When I am trying to get the ball away from an opposing woman, they maneuver around me as if I were a statue. Plus I keep fouling everybody. I jam two fingers the first week. The next week I get there early and practice shooting. My friend shows me how she flicks her wrist to get proper rotation on the ball and this helps me make some baskets. We go over the rules so I won't foul as much. She tells me that when I am on defense, I should watch the stomach of the woman I am guarding, this way I will know which way she will turn. When the other women come we begin playing, and several mention how much I have improved. I glow a thousand times more than I ever did after being told I was pretty.

Competitive sports, I learned, are transcendent. When you are in the game, you forget everything—work, stress, that your boyfriend is mad at you. None of it matters. Time itself is altered, and you ride above it in a zone where everything is good. Two hours of soccer go by and I don't even notice. I am exercising without exercising.

I start playing tennis, because I've always wanted to, and because the Williams sisters (Venus and Serena) are really, really cool. Upon a friend's recommendation, I start with lessons, learn how to hold the racket and hit the ball. When I get it right, it feels fluid and natural. I am rallying with my instructor and hit one right down the line, out of his reach. I clench my fists, secretly pretending I have won a championship point. Soon I play with a friend who started lessons when she was five. The way she serves and hits the ball looks so graceful I want to sneak away while she's not looking. I am way out of my league and lose 6-0, 6-1. I consider the single game won an accomplishment.

This year I plan to try hockey, racquetball, and skiing. In the meantime, between soccer, basketball, and tennis, I am in the greatest shape of my life. Soccer is the highlight—I can't wait for Saturdays. Last week I ran to tackle someone, to kick the ball away from them, but I skidded and came down on my hands and knees. After the game we sat in the park and stretched and I looked at the blood clotting. In the way a smell can evoke a memory, the sight and feel of my skinned knees transported me. Suddenly I am eleven years old, running after a soccer ball coming toward our goal. Ryan, the little twerp, gets to it first and kicks it ahead, setting up for an easy goal. I lunge, skidding my feet just ahead of him, kicking the ball away. Then we play dodge ball and I get him out on the first throw. The recess bell rings. I win.

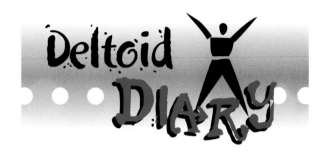

Deltoid DIARY

Auto Pilates

When I walked into the Body Tech Shop in one of the ritzier parts of the city, I didn't know what to expect. I figured that Pilates, the stretching and toning technique dancers use to lengthen and strengthen muscles, was similar to yoga. It has received a lot of hype because gorgeous celebrities like Uma Thurman and Sharon Stone practice it. Those who swear by it say that it will give you a nice streamlined look, similar to that of a ballerina. I could go for that.

However, in my mind I didn't see how it was different from any other stretching class. It looked like yoga's more glamorous cousin.

At the gym, I found my exercise instructor, Ean (pronounced Ean), pacing in a dimmed room with mirrored walls. So I asked him if I was in for upscale yoga. "No," he said with the patient look you have when a five-year-old asks a question. "It's not quite like anything else."

Since I was new to the class and it showed, Ean took the opportunity to explain to me how to breathe the Pilates way. Pilates, developed in the 1920s by Joseph Pilates, teaches that if you breathe properly and control your movements, the exercise will help lengthen and strengthen the body, including your spine. In order to breathe Pilates-style, I put my hands under my ribcage and inhaled while pushing my ribcage out.

"Exhale," he said, "by pushing the air out with a loud hissing noise." It felt backwards, so I tried taking several Pilates breaths before class began.

I grabbed a mat and a long rubbery band, which Ean said would help me in the class. After the class took a few breaths in unison, he had us lie down on our backs while slowly swinging our legs from side to side. We bent our knees and flexed our feet as he instructed us through the routine. He also told us when to breathe in and out. You'd think breathing would come fairly naturally, but when it came to breathing the Pilates way while bending, pointing, and flexing, it wasn't that simple.

Next came another pose in which we moved onto our stomachs with outstretched arms and legs, sort of like seals. I quickly felt how this movement could align the body because I felt a full stretch in my stomach, arms, and legs.

Like good pets, we next rolled on our backs, lifted a leg into a 90 degree angle, and swung it in a controlled movement to the left and circled it to the right. I got the left swing okay, but Ean had to come over and manually circle my leg for me. My brain said, "circle," but my leg didn't listen.

As I learned, the movements in Pilates feel very different from yoga, mainly because there are fewer contortions. My muscles seemed to fatigue at some points but they never hurt. I felt stretched in areas of my body I didn't know would stretch.

The most challenging part of the Pilates class was undoubtedly the controlled rocks. We sat in a position similar to Indian-style with our backs slightly curved. Next, we rolled onto our backs and sat up in the same position without our feet touching the ground. I could roll back okay, but I couldn't seem to get back up. Ean looked sympathetically as I struggled into an upright position. "This is the hardest pose," he said, advising me to round my back more. (Now I know how a turtle feels.)

In Pilates, you are cautioned to back off if your body rejects a move. I was on my way to rejecting the rolls, when the hour was up. We completed at least 10 poses in the class. When Ean told us to stand up and breathe (I had gotten better at the Pilates breathing by then), I felt as if I was standing straighter. I really could feel that my posture had improved and I certainly felt as if I had worked out. The best thing about Pilates is that since the movements are slow and controlled, you don't have to worry about overexertion.

However, it's not very likely that you will lose a ton of weight. Because it is said to lengthen the muscles, you will appear slimmer if you practice Pilates correctly and stick with it about three times a week. You might not look like a ballerina, but at least you might feel like one.

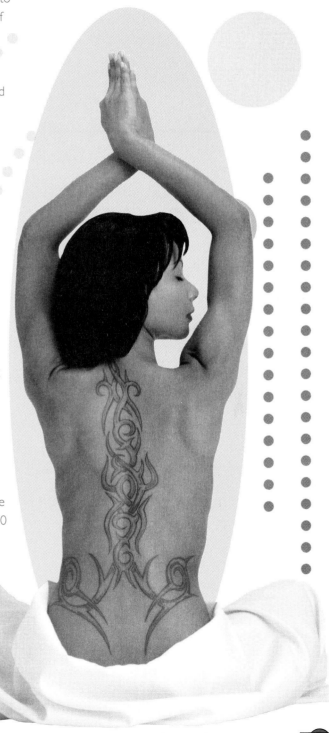

9 ONE FRANTIC FITNESS

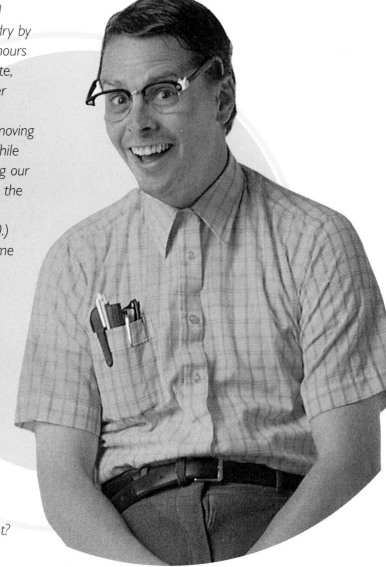

What is it that they say about "good intentions?" That they get sucked dry by mindless TV and frozen dinners, late-night hours and overtime, the rat race and the commute, the vending machine and the movie theater concession stand? Or something like that.

What is true is that most people are moving at a much faster pace than ever before. While technology and the Internet may be making our lives easier, they're not adding any hours to the day. (Although, Bill Gates might still have something up his sleeve for Windows 2010.) But for now, we're still working more overtime and driving longer commutes.

Naturally, all of this rushing here and there has a negative effect on our daily workouts and healthy diets. Is it always convenient to pack a plastic baggie full of carrot slices for lunch in the morning? Or is it easier to just grab a pack of Ring Dings from the commissary vending machine? And do you really feel like heading off to the gym at 8 p.m. after another long day at work when Die Hard: The Geriatric Years is playing in the Supermultiplex across the street?

Popcorn still counts as a vegetable, right?

WORKPLACE WORKOUTS, OR: SWEATIN' TO THE MUZAC

Excuses, excuses! Everybody yearns to get in better shape, yet most working people find it difficult to set aside the time for an adequate workout. According to the U.S. Census, people are working longer hours and traveling farther to work. And according to the American Medical Association, Americans are growing fatter and exercising less. Coincidence? Doubtful.

How do you fit a workout into a busy work and commute schedule, especially if you want to have some time to spend with your friends? The good news is, you don't necessarily have to free up an hour of exercise time during your work day. You can still reap the benefits of physical activity in short spurts of five to 15 minutes at a time.

EXERCISING WHILE YOU COMMUTE

Think about all the time you spend sitting on your butt just getting to and from work.

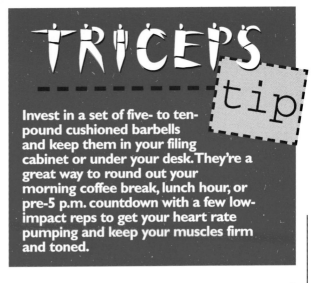

Reaching for your cappuccino or cell phone doesn't count as exercise, but burning calories doesn't have to be much more complicated than that.

The simplest way to work exercise into your commute is to do part of your traveling by foot or bicycle. If you normally drive to the train station, bus stop, or park-and-ride lot, why not walk or ride your bike? Bike racks can be found at most transit points, and some even have bicycle lockers.

Believe it or not, there are also exercises you can do in your seat on the train or bus. Some can even be

TRICEPS tip

Invest in a set of five- to ten-pound cushioned barbells and keep them in your filing cabinet or under your desk. They're a great way to round out your morning coffee break, lunch hour, or pre-5 p.m. countdown with a few low-impact reps to get your heart rate pumping and keep your muscles firm and toned.

done while you're driving a car (but if you are talking on your cell phone and eating a donut, you're increasing your degree of difficulty significantly). These exercises combine stretching and isometrics (tensing a muscle and holding it in a stationary position while maintaining the tension). Squeeze balls or rubber resistance bands can easily fit in a purse or briefcase. If you feel foolish as other people look at you in your car doing *something* that definitely does not look like adjusting the radio, just smile back with a very satisfied look and flex your bulging arm muscles. That should do it.

EXERCISING IN
THE OFFICE

Once you arrive in the office, you should be nicely warmed up. Of course, work is secondary, so you look for the next logical opportunity for exercise, such as a coffee break, in between tasks, or lunch.

A good course would be to take a brisk 20-minute walk outside.

Walking can be done anywhere, doesn't require any special equipment, and the fresh air and change of surroundings can be therapeutic after avoiding as much work as possible. Make sure you have a pair of walking shoes that fit well with plenty of support. Start slowly to warm up, but then try to maintain an energetic pace. You can also incorporate light hand weights for some toning. Here's a trick: Use two small water bottles—one in each hand—as hand weights. By the time you're done, you should have finished the water in both bottles. During your walk, don't stop and start but keep walking without pause for as long as your schedule allows. You can devise various routes that you know will take about 20 minutes from start to finish.

If your job involves sitting at a desk for long periods of time, seize every opportunity to get up and move around. (You'll earn the nickname Mr. Fidget, but it's worth it.) Take the stairs whenever possible. Instead of visiting a rest room on your floor, walk up several flights of stairs to another floor. Offer to hoist the bottled water into the cooler (remember to bend at the knees). Take the long way around the cubicle farm to see your coworkers.

Avoid the convenient temptation of vending machines and keep healthy snacks, such as fruit and nuts, at your desk. Keep a bottle of water on your desk at all times. This will cut down on your calorie intake.

CHAPTER 9: FRANTIC FITNESS

When you get up to put a file away, take a few minutes to stretch. Do a few shoulder rolls. Let your arms hang

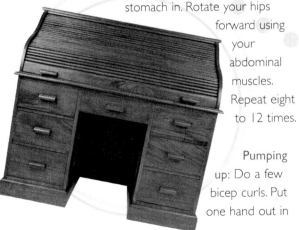

relaxed at your sides. As you inhale, bring your shoulders forward, then up, exhale as you bring them back, then down. Imagine you're drawing a big circle with your shoulders. Do this four times. Then reverse the circle. Shoulders back, then up, then forward, and down. Be sure to breathe while doing this exercise. Do it slowly and relaxed.

If your job makes you a slave to your desk, such as a receptionist, there are still exercises you can do without ever leaving your post. A chair and a desk are just about the only equipment required for these workouts, and there's no need to change clothes, provided your outfit allows for freedom of movement. Do these whenever you have a spare minute, such as waiting for a document to print or holding for someone on the phone. What are you waiting for?

Crunch: To strengthen your abdominals, sit with your back straight. Rotate your hips back, curling your stomach in. Rotate your hips forward using your abdominal muscles. Repeat eight to 12 times.

Pumping up: Do a few bicep curls. Put one hand out in front of you, palm up. This is your curling arm. Put your other hand on the wrist of your curling arm. Press down with your top hand to provide resistance, while you raise your bottom hand up. Imagine you're curling a weight. Repeat eight to 12 times, then switch arms.

Kick up your heels with leg curls: Place your hands on the desk for support. Extend one leg out behind you, not to the side. Bend your knee

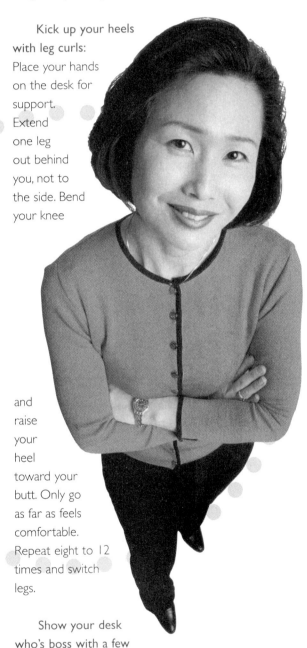

and raise your heel toward your butt. Only go as far as feels comfortable. Repeat eight to 12 times and switch legs.

Show your desk who's boss with a few push-ups: Stand a few feet away from your desk. Put your hands on the desk, shoulder width apart. Keep your back straight. Lower your chest toward the desk, then push out. Don't rush. Repeat eight to 12 times.

The result: Soon people in your office will note that you are a mass of nervous energy, and they'll probably recommend counseling. But at least you'll look good for your therapist.

CORPORATE WELLNESS PROGRAMS

Many companies are taking a more active role in promoting the health of their employees, offering health care screenings, weight management classes, nutrition programs, and on-site fitness centers.

Quality wellness programs reduce health care costs, make employees more productive, and reduce workplace stress. Some companies have onsite fitness centers with exercise machines, free weights, aerobics and exercise classes, and outdoor walking or jogging paths.

If you're lucky enough to work for such an employer, take full advantage of this benefit. You will be much more likely to stick with an exercise program if you can fit it in at the work site, either before or after work, or during a lunch break. Most programs are heavily subsidized to keep the monthly fees minimal. Think of the freedom you'll feel at arriving home with your workout behind you and an evening ahead when you can be a total vegetable.

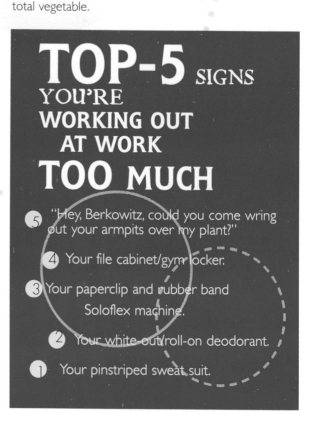

TOP-5 SIGNS
YOU'RE
**WORKING OUT
AT WORK
TOO MUCH**

5 "Hey, Berkowitz, could you come wring out your armpits over my plant?"

4 Your file cabinet/gym locker.

3 Your paperclip and rubber band Soloflex machine.

2 Your white-out/roll-on deodorant.

1 Your pinstriped sweat suit.

DINING IN TONIGHT, SIR?
VENDING MACHINE MENU,
OR: YOU HAVE MUNCHIE MADNESS

Vending machines. Ah, sweet relief. Whether you raid them for your breakfast each morning (B-3), for dessert after lunch (A-4), or for that all important mid-afternoon snack (F-6), vending machines can mean the difference between a sweet sugar high or a low sugar attack.

But when's the last time you saw something healthy hanging in your vending machine?

What's that? Listen, pal, just because Slim Jim sounds like a diet aid, that doesn't mean that long slab of processed meat stuff is fat-free. And no, Fig Newtons don't exactly qualify as a serving of fruits and vegetables, either. But don't fret, a trip to the vending machine doesn't have to set your fitness program back a notch. Just follow these helpful tips to make vending machines a little less villainous.

BREAK YOUR ROUTINE

Just because you have your vending machine favorites memorized in order of sweetness to salty ratio (try A-6 first, if that's out, go for B-2, if that's out, try F-8, etc.) it doesn't mean those are the only three buttons on the entire machine. Look past your nose at those chips hanging in the forty-five cent row, or the pastries down at the bottom for seventy-five cents. There could be healthy options you're overlooking.

THE WORST OF THE WORST

Here are your choices: Cheese–peanut butter crackers, potato chips, fat-free cookies, sourdough pretzel nuggets, chocolate mini-donuts, pretzel twists, microwave popcorn, animal crackers, fat-free chocolate sandwich cookies, and frosted Pop-Tarts. Hmm, skip the chips and Pop-Tarts right away. Most bags of chips, potato, nacho, or otherwise, can often contain up to 250+ calories and 15+ grams of fat. And Pop-Tarts, even if you toast them (no the heat does not "burn" calories), they're still up to 400 calories and up to 10 grams of fat. And the chocolate donuts? Forget about it. Read the label and, when you pick yourself back up off the floor, put them and their 800 calories back in the slot for some other sucker!

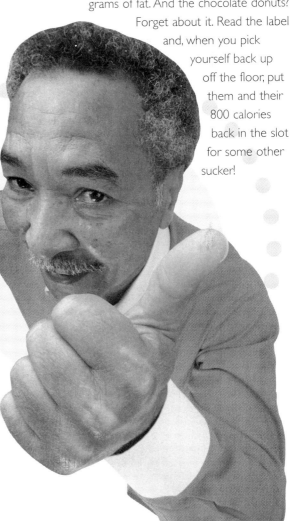

TRICEPS tip

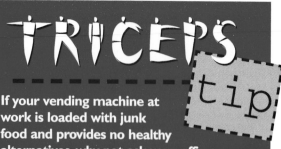

If your vending machine at work is loaded with junk food and provides no healthy alternatives, why not ask your office manager when the vending machine representative comes. Meet him at the machine and make a few healthy suggestions. Chances are, he doesn't get too many and will gladly switch out at least one or two items to keep his healthy customers happy. Repay him by choosing those selections, or reminding coworkers that they are now there.

raisins? Sure. These deceiving little snack crackers are usually high in calories (a mere six contain 210 calories), loaded with fat (the saturated kind), and contain just a single gram of fiber.

What's the biggest "worst of the worst" surprise: How about those fat-free cookies? Sure, the name of the company may be Healthy something or other, and there's enough blaring fat-free labels covering the package to send you into advertising shock. But these little morsels often contain just as many calories as their fat-full companions, because they substitute sugar for the fat!

Microwave popcorn may seem like a pretty good bet, but unless it says "light," these bags of popcorn fun can contain up to 400 calories per bag! Okay then, what about those nuclear day-glo orange cheese–peanut butter crackers? People munch them all the time at work. They can't be bad, right?

THE BEST OF THE BEST

Corn chips, nacho chips, potato chips, pretzels, cheese crackers, salted peanuts, chocolate mini-donuts, shortbread cookies, chewing gum, and hard candies. Hmm, which sweet or salty snack in this munchie mine field does the least damage? Actually, you have several choices. After all, just because you were wearing diapers the last time you tried animal crackers doesn't mean they're still hanging around for nothing. These lion and monkey shaped gems are generally low in calories and saturated fat. (Many packages even boast "2 grams of fat per bag.") And why not? As far as snack foods go, that's pretty darn good.

What else? How about pretzels? Generally low in calories and containing little or no fat, they're filling,

Well, define "bad." As bad as 800 calories worth of chocolate covered donuts? No. Worse than a nice apple and a box of crunchy, and don't leave orange nuclear dust all over your keyboard. Sure, they're a little salty, but that's what water coolers are for. For a runner-up, try salted peanuts. Sure, nuts get a bad rep, but the tiny size they give you in the vending machine makes a filling, high-protein alternative to many other choices.

But what about something for your sweet tooth? Hit the button for chewing gum. Not only is it one of the cheapest items in the vending machine, but it gives you the sweetness you want without the fat or the calories.

LUCKY SUCKERS

If you're lucky enough, you work in an office that has a fresh-food vending machine. (If you just took off your John Deere cap, scratched your noodle, and said, "Huh? What you mean by fresh?" then we're not talking to you.) These revolving door contraptions, similar to those pictured in 1950-era cafeterias, are refrigerated and often contain such healthful samplings as skim milk, V8 juice, canned "light" fruit cocktail, instant noodle soup cup, yogurt, plain bagel with cream cheese, green salad (dressing on the side), chicken-salad sandwich, ham and cheese sandwich, and even a baked potato topped with broccoli and cheddar cheese.

Start with the skim milk. It's a rich source of calcium and protein, low in saturated fat and cholesterol, and eight ounces contains only 90 calories. Other great choices are the salad, the yogurt, or the V8 juice. Avoid the sandwiches altogether (unless you're trapped in the office for dinner) and only eat the baked potato if you scrape off the cheese first.

BEVERAGE CART

Fruit punch, cranberry-raspberry blend, cranberry juice, orange juice, water, berry lemonade, sports drink, apple juice, or iced tea. Cola, diet cola, cherry cola, root beer, orange soda, ginger ale, or plain seltzer. While vending machines are generally all the same, what goes inside can be as varied as a Snickers bar and a bag of jalapeño pork rinds. Cold drink machines are no different. And, while many folks consider the drink machine a mere appetizer or side dish for the pièce de resistance, the snack machine, the right choice in beverage could be a fitting substitute for what hangs in the dreaded snack machine.

So let's start with the healthiest first: Water. It's pure, it's natural, and it's calorie-free. Besides, thanks to coffee and tea, not to mention sodas and those sugary "juice beverages," we often need more of it than we usually get. Water quenches thirst, which may be mistaken for hunger. Of course, you could get a drink from the office fountain for free. (But we know you like to look cool, and there's nothing cooler than spending a dollar on a chilly bottle of H2O.)

What's next? Try plain seltzer, if it's available. It has much of the same strengths as water, plus the added fun and pizazz of bubbles! Okay, water and seltzer are fine, but you're a little hungry, not just thirsty. No doubt about it, try 100-percent orange juice or apple juice.

Both come in cans these days, and can make a nice after-noon snack all by themselves, or round out a more fulfilling snack of pretzels or nuts. Just make

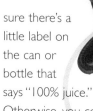

sure there's a little label on the can or bottle that says "100% juice." Otherwise, you could end up drinking an expensive bottle of colored sugar water flavored like oranges or apples.

Okay, okay. Water's great and juice is sweet, but you crave sugar. Well, if the fruit juices aren't sweet enough, diet colas can often be mistaken for sweet and temporarily curb your sweet tooth, but so can iced tea. Make sure it's unsweetened, and then snag a sugar substitute from the coffee condiment rack and add it yourself. And, while it's pushing it to call ginger ale a "health food," it can calm an empty stomach, and it's lower in sugar than some sodas.

So what's the worst? Actually, it's a toss-up between soda and juice. Sweet sodas are full of sugar and can often be just as full of calories as a candy bar or pastry from the snack machine. And "juice drinks" may sound healthy, and even have healthful pictures of fruit just bursting with healthiness on the can or bottle, but the average serving contains 110 calories—and there's often two per bottle!—the highest in this group. Also, any time a beverage is labeled "blend" or "ade" or "drink," it often has less than 5 percent fruit juice inside. (Translated: You'd get just as much juice if you squeezed a lime into your Schweppes seltzer!)

OVERTIME DINNERTIME

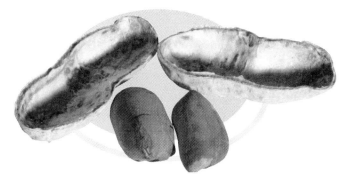

Unfortunately, it's not uncommon to find yourself looking up from your besieged desk and seeing that it's dark outside your porthole-sized office window. So what do you do for dinner when it's too late to pile a heavy meal on an empty stomach or you don't have time to actually step foot out of your office building and try to find a fast food place?

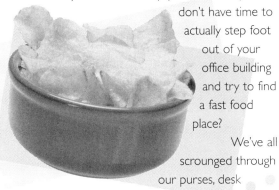

We've all scrounged through our purses, desk drawers, and even a coworker's desk drawer who's gone home for the night. (You snoop!) And so, armed with enough change to fill one of those god awful Crown Royal bags, we trudge down to the break room, wave to the custodians, and attempt to find a reasonable dinner from the hanging bags of chips, cookies, and pastries.

So what should you choose that won't send you flying on a sugar high or emptying the water cooler over your mouth to alleviate a salt overdose? Actually, you have two pretty good choices which, not by coincidence we're sure, are also two of the most popular items in vending machines across the land.

One option is to choose those cheese–peanut butter crackers, especially if your drink machine offers skim milk as a side dish. "But wait!" you gasp. Yes, yes, we know. You just read that cheese crackers were one of the worst snack foods. But this is different. This is dinner. And, since a "meal" (we use the term loosely here) should be between 350 and 600 calories and contain enough fat to tide you over to the next meal, cheese crackers certainly fit the bill. (If you can't quite stomach the thought of orange crackers and processed peanut butter synthetic spread grease as dinner, opt for a couple of bags of peanuts and wash them down with apple juice.)

If you don't want to digest all of the saturated fat found in peanuts, however, why not go for a bag or two of the pretzels and one bag of peanuts? Yes, it's a salty combination, but it also combines carbohydrates, protein, and mono-unsaturated fat. To stave off a thirst attack, drink a glass or two of water to compensate for the sodium you've taken in.

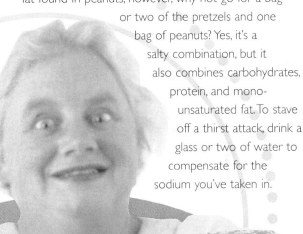

DESSERT, ANYONE?

As if there weren't enough choices for you to make at your local vending machine (gee, who knew snack time could be as much work as, well, work?), what's for dessert? Okay, you know better than to reach for the donuts or sweet rolls, Pop Tarts or pastries. But what about candy bars? And what's with all these new energy bars, anyway?

Read the labels on a few samples of each, however, and you'll find that, ounce for ounce, candy and energy bars have about the same number of calories. (Often in the 250+ range, no less.) However, it's the amount of fat, including saturated fat, that can really add up in a simple candy bar, often to the tune of twice as high in a chocolate candy bar. Although energy bars do contain vitamins, minerals, and some dietary fiber, most are simply snazzed up candy bars with a few extras thrown in to qualify for federal label laws. Sort of like adding vitamins to

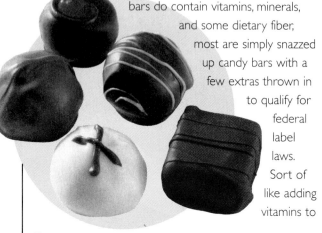

Cap'n Crunch or Frosted Flakes and calling them Healthy Choice cereals.

However, both bars have their uses. For instance, if you don't have time to go out and grab some take-out or even have something delivered, some of the more substantial (and expensive) energy bars can come in handy. Those labeled "nutritional supplements," for instance, contain vitamins and minerals, unlike a candy bar, and can be quite substantial when paired with a glass of milk or juice.

Also, if you're on your way to the gym and don't have the time to eat a full meal and then wait for it to digest, try having one of the lighter, low-fat, energy bars, one with about 150 calories, and eat it in the car.

So, when exactly is it acceptable to eat a candy bar? Well, for starters: You can eat candy bars for

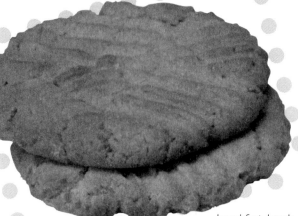

breakfast, lunch, and dinner, not to mention every hour on the hour in between, if you feel like it that is, and aren't too fond of your teeth. However, for the purposes of a book on exercise and fitness that is trying to help you feel as good as possible about yourself, there are actually a few cases where a candy bar can come in handy.

For instance, if you are having an undeniable craving for chocolate, a candy bar is a much better bet than an energy bar. Candy bars tend to be smaller than energy bars, so you don't have to pretend that you're going to eat just half. Also, candy bars are a lot cheaper than their snootier cousins, those energy bars, and if you choose the right ones, such as a candy bar filled with nuts, you'll at least get some protein and fiber. So what the heck. Go for it!

EATING (TOO MUCH) OUT

The cupboards are bare. The refrigerator contains only a half-eaten container of yogurt with an expiration date that's soon to have its one-year anniversary. And both you and your significant other are so haggard from work that the stack of dirty dishes overflowing from the sink seems a more momentous challenge than climbing Mt. Everest in a thong. We've all had these nights. You and your partner look deep into each other's eyes and ask the obvious question simultaneously: "Where do you want to eat?"

Let's face it, people today are busier than ever before. With both parents working coupled with longer hours and, in many cases, longer commutes, eating out becomes a very enticing option. Just open the Yellow Pages

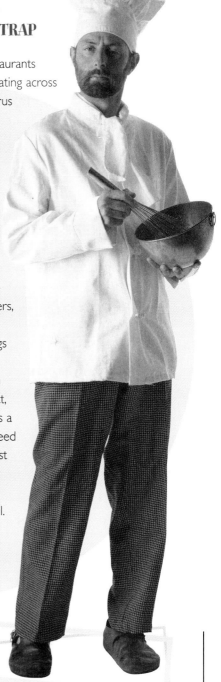

to "Restaurant" and your eyes will bug out from all the possible dining experiences you and your family can delight in. There is Chinese, Italian, Russian, Indian, Thai, Japanese, Ethiopian, Mediterranean, and, of course, good old American cuisine to choose from.

That's only the tip of the iceberg! But as you and your significant other go about selecting a place to satiate your hunger pains—an ordeal that could take hours—keep in mind the desires of your taste buds and time constraints can make even the most steadfast dieter forget the waist line they're trying to shrink.

THE FAST FOOD TRAP

Fast food restaurants have been proliferating across the states like a virus since the 1950s. Today, there are over 300,000 fast food restaurants in the U.S. alone, all contributing to obesity and heart disease every day. The food they serve—those cheeseburgers, boxes of chicken wings, and hot dogs on a stick—are notoriously high in calories, sodium, fat, and cholesterol. It's a diet that's guaranteed to thicken the waist and cause massive heart attacks if a person isn't careful.

Foods high in fat—like most fast food—can cause hardening of the arteries, coronary heart disease, and stroke. There is also an increased chance of developing breast and colon cancer when consuming fatty foods. This is something to keep in mind the next time you and a friend are waiting in a drive-thru. Have a conversation about it. Maybe your friend doesn't know that burger he's going to eat will clog the plumbing in his heart or cause tumors to grow inside his lower intestine. Remember that real friends don't let friends get colon cancer.

However, if you can't resist the temptation of quick food that you can eat while driving, ordering cautiously at the drive-thru can still be very beneficial. Instead of ordering a quarter-pound burger with cheese, order a plain old hamburger. Instead of super-sizing your French fries, order small fries. Instead of a nine-piece box of chicken nuggets, order a six-piece. It's amazing how fast all those calories add up. Just trim down the extras.

SALLY'S
TECHNIQUE

In the movie *When Harry Met Sally . . .*, Meg Ryan's character was always very specific when she ordered her food at a restaurant. She knew what she wanted and how she wanted it prepared. Although this characteristic became a comic effect in the film, there is nothing wrong with telling your waiter exactly how you want your food. They are there to serve the customer. If they give you a hassle or a dirty look, maybe they don't

want a tip. This is something to keep in mind while you're trying to diet or maintain a health regimen. If you don't want butter on your toast, just say so before the temptation is sitting before you, calling out "eat me!"

A good idea is to order foods that are light to begin with, that way you don't have to worry about fattening ingredients. Salads, for instance, are always a light option so long as you don't smother them in thick, creamy dressings like Ranch or Thousand Island. A good way to scrap dressing altogether is to order lemon wedges on the side and squeeze some lemon juice on the salad. Lemons are a great condiment (and for more than just vodka tonics).

However, there will undoubtedly be times when you must have that certain dish—that certain fatty dish—that makes you bloat just by looking at it. A string of drool falls from your mouth onto the picture in the menu. You must have it. But it's so fattening. What to do? Just remember Sally's technique in *When Harry Met Sally . . . .* Look at the dish and tell the waiter what you don't want included. Don't be shy! If they spit in your food, it's one hell of a lucrative lawsuit.

Here are a few examples of how to order carefully.

PIZZA!

Your friends want to order a pizza. Instead of piling on a mountain of toppings, choose the ingredients wisely. A meat lover's pizza, for instance, is begging for disaster. Vegetarian pizzas, on the other hand, are an excellent way to avoid excessive fat and calories. Some people also ask pizza parlors to hold the cheese. This may sound disgusting, but it is a necessary evil if you're truly trying to slim down. Cheese is the arch enemy of all dieters!

GRILLED SALMON AND POTATOES

Restaurants will use oils to grill salmon, chicken, and beef even if they advertise themselves as organic and healthy. But this shouldn't stop you from enjoying a splurge. These very same restaurants will be glad to grill your salmon without oil. They will also, if requested, substitute those buttery potatoes with an extra side of steamed vegetables. The result of this conscientious treat will be a delicious meal without the worry of busting the scale in the morning.

ANYTHING IN SAUCE

Sauces can make a meal delicious just as effectively as they can make a waist wide. Who doesn't like Alfredo on their pasta or a wine sauce smothering their entree? But sauces, no matter how appetizing they are, must be sacrificed. A steak, already detrimental to a healthy diet, is twice as villainous when bathing in a pool of béarnaise sauce. And noodles are much more healthy when covered with vegetables than when they're drowned in a creamy white or a chunky red sauce. Whatever you order make sure it's *sans* sauce.

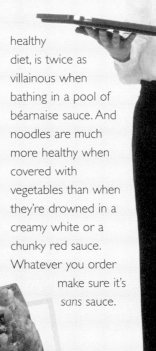

APPETIZERS & DESSERTS? HA!

Appetizers are designed to whet people's appetites. But, if you survey friends and your own memory, you'll discover that most people are unbearably full after their salad, soup, or roasted garlic platter. The first course is the most satisfying part of any meal, without a doubt. It delivers us from our misery of hunger so that we can savor our dinner. But for all their good points, appetizers can be one excess too many. That order of nachos or jalapeño poppers can nullify any attempts at a diet. It's tempting—oh so very tempting—but you must resist. Similarly, once you've finished your dinner and the waiter offers the dessert menu, the devil on your shoulder will undoubtedly yell in your ear, "Order the Banana Split!" There will be many appealing pictures on the menu. Ice cream covered in hot fudge! Cheesecake in a caramel sauce. A slice of chocolate cake with whipped cream and a cherry on top. It'll be unbearable to look at. It will be painful to deny yourself. But you must say "no!" All the careful ordering you did at dinner will be for naught if you don't.

BE STRONG!

Going out to dinner is a treat to begin with, so you must be all the more committed to your diet. It's easy to get caught up in the moment and say, "Well, we're having this treat so why not forget this damn diet for one night." It's only natural. But the next day, you'll be kicking yourself for sure. "What was I thinking? I'm so weak!"

Don't put yourself in this situation. When you sit down at the table, resist any temptation to throw caution to the wind. Acknowledge that there are things you want, you crave, you desire, but continually remind yourself of your goal. Pat yourself on the back every time you make a wise choice. Hey, self-righteousness can be fun.

TIME (MIS) MANAGEMENT

If you remain serious about working out for an extended period of time, you're bound to notice what should have been obvious but was probably overlooked: 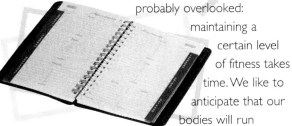 maintaining a certain level of fitness takes time. We like to anticipate that our bodies will run themselves once we set them on the right the course. That would be a just reward for working so hard in the first place.

And to some degree, that's what happens: A week off from running is not as large a setback for a highly trained athlete as it is for the beginning jogger. But a running routine in either case is still a serious time suck. You can easily find it hard to manage your time to continually include a workout routine.

TIME MANAGEMENT IS PRIORITY MANAGEMENT

Your free time choices reflect what is important to you. Someone who works overtime every weekend obviously has different priorities than someone who is out sailing with his buddies or traveling with her family. Fitness can be another priority that you may choose to include in your free time choices. If you're more interested in being in shape than you are in

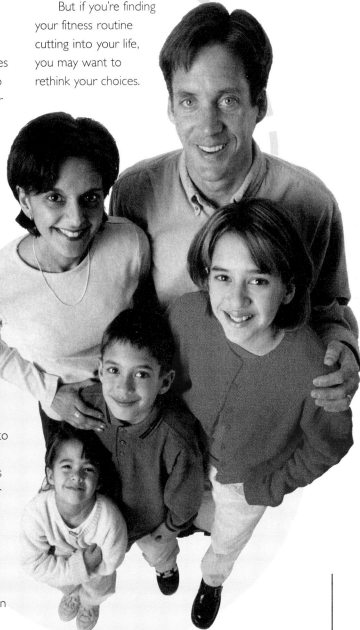

prime-time television, choose to hit the gym after work for two hours each night instead.

Your free time management, though, may not exactly reflect the priorities that you think you hold. If your family is most important to you, but working out is cutting into your time with them, there's a tension that will probably need to be resolved. You may be lucky enough that they are sympathetic and understanding. Or you may be justified because your choices are temporary—you're on a short-term training schedule, for example.

But if you're finding your fitness routine cutting into your life, you may want to rethink your choices.

Unless a huge bench press really is more important than a happy husband or significant other, then you may eventually adjust your free time management so that it reflects your actual priorities.

Similar consideration may be in order if your workouts begin to jeopardize your work. If nobody cares that you leave at 4:45 every day to make it to the early spinning class, than all the better for you and your quads. But if you find yourself leaving projects half-finished or being unprepared at the next morning's meeting because you cut out early, you may want to adjust your schedule. Again, you may be the lucky guy with the sympathetic office environment. If your boss respects your choices and makes allowances for your early departure, then small adjustments may be all that's needed to get your work back on track.

If, on the other hand, you find yourself being glared at as you leave—and especially if you feel your job is threatened or you're losing out on benefits like a promotion—the later spinning class may be the better choice. While your priorities are always your own decision, you can't pay for a gym membership if you don't earn a salary.

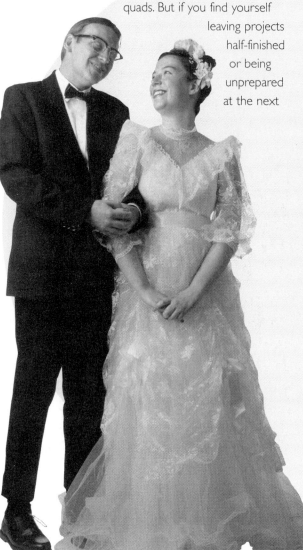

SNEAKY TRAPS

If you're like most fitness freaks, you're not really about to sacrifice your relationships or your job for the gym—you're sure you would never let a situation get that bad. But you can mismanage your time in less obvious ways, by compromising the quality of the time you commit to other things. If you are so tired from working out that you nearly fall asleep during a dinner date, you may not be any better than the girl who skips the dinner date entirely so that she can go to the gym.

If you keep dozing during dates, you may even stop making them entirely, since you expect to be too tired. Once you find yourself sacrificing quality, you are probably on the way to serious time mismanagement. That's because if you keep doing something (like dating) badly, you'll probably decide not to do it at all. A lonely muscle-bound future is no better than a scrawny one.

If you are one of those hyper-scheduled people who lives for her Filofax, you can expect your anal ways to carry over to your fitness routine. Do you jot down which exercises you should do each day, so that you know at the beginning of the month how many bicep workouts you can expect to fit in?

And do you also write down your weekly Kickboxing class, even though the time never changes? (Can you say "obsession"???) Unfortunately, this kind of maintenance can make for particularly deadly time mismanagement. It can be key to keeping a long-term commitment to fitness.

But it can be overdone. Once you write something down, you are more inclined to do it. So if you're scheduled to lift from 7 to 9, then your significant other is just going to have to wait to eat dinner. Every night. Even on the days that he can't. You can imagine that this sort of mismanagement is bound to end badly.

Been there? Done that? Does this sound like you: You've demanded bitchily and begged shamelessly until every person you cared about was rearranging their schedules around your workout routine. Hmm, not very fair to your friends and family, is it? And, most likely, it wasn't a particularly nice reflection of

your priorities. The gym is important, and scheduling is one of the reasons that you've remained so faithful to your workout. But it's always open tomorrow. And it's got some of the longest hours around. And dinner at 10 just plain sucks.

SEMI-EXCEPTIONS

There's a time and a place to be a hard-ass about your workout schedule. But there's also got to be a reason. One of the best reasons to be strict about your routine is that your routine is particularly strict—perhaps because you're training for a particular event, like a contest or marathon.

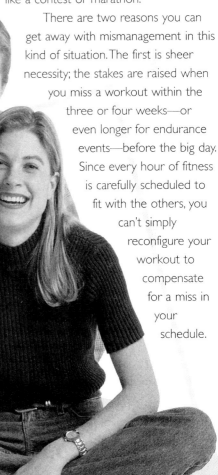

There are two reasons you can get away with mismanagement in this kind of situation. The first is sheer necessity; the stakes are raised when you miss a workout within the three or four weeks—or even longer for endurance events—before the big day. Since every hour of fitness is carefully scheduled to fit with the others, you can't simply reconfigure your workout to compensate for a miss in your schedule.

tip

If you can't seem to find the time to exercise regularly, try an abbreviated workout when time is tight. The key is increasing the intensity to compensate for the reduced duration.

Perhaps more important, there is a defined end date for this kind of commitment. After you bench press 300 pounds for charity, you're not going to want to pick up a weight for a few weeks anyway.

And after keeping to a gruelingly tight schedule for the month preceding a tri-state bike race, you're probably going to naturally cut yourself a break from training. The New York Roadrunner's Club, who organizes the New York City Marathon, calls the collective time mismanagement that comes with marathon training "ATM disease," and cautions runners to limit how often they begin a sentence with "After the Marathon."

Another reason that you may want to tighten your gym schedule is that you're having a hard time finding any time for it at all. The holidays are one common

example; between the office party on Tuesday, the shopping that you need to do on Wednesday, and your parents flying in on Thursday, you don't have the time to put up the decorations let alone a decent set of military presses.

In this case, it may be necessary—both logistically and emotionally—to block out a time that you are committed to working out. Again, this only works because it comes with an expiration date, often sometime at the end of December. And, really, it's probably better for you to take care of yourself and your body for an hour one night than to miserably eat pounds of cocktail wieners out of obligation.

IF YOU CAN'T QUIT

If you find yourself struggling with tension between fitness and other commitments, the most mature decision is probably to scale back your workouts. As should be clear by now, time management is priority management. So, if working out is less important than your relationships or your livelihood, than it should take a back burner to these things when they get hot.

The mature decision, however, is rarely the fun one, and that irony certainly applies to working out. Every exercise enthusiast has been there: You know full well that it's a bad idea to cut out of work at 4:00 on a Wednesday with the Munsen project due on Friday, but you would just rather be lifting than researching. Who wouldn't choose to work up a sweat over working up another fifty-page report? Exercise feels good, which makes it addictive. There are some sneaky strategies you can employ when you need your fix.

Above all else, you need to think outside the box when it comes to scheduling your time. Who says you need to work on the Munsen project from 9 to noon and 1 to 5 every day? If you must report your clocked time, then think about bringing your lunch and working through that hour so that you can get out of work and into the gym earlier. The bonus: Few people take advantage of this possibility, so you'll have your run of equipment instead of waiting for someone else's half hour on the treadmill to run out. If sneaking out early might still provoke eyebrows, think about taking a chunk out of the middle of your day.

One of the world's biggest management consulting groups expects its employees to take two hours in the middle of their day, so that they can break up the long hours that they must work.

Quite a few of those yuppies use that time for a run, while the sun is still shining and before they're tired from a full day of work. The American workplace is being flexed, slowly but surely. Thanks to the efforts of mothers, in particular, most bosses understand that workers want to reconfigure the 9 to 5 workday in order to best address their other life priorities. It might be perfectly appropriate for you to suggest that your physical health is similarly important to you.

If you find your workouts compromising your relationships with family or friends, then you might hope that they are the ones who rethink things. Wouldn't it be perfect if they started joining you? That way, you wouldn't have to choose between your best friend and your leg workout. Really, it's win-win if you can get your boyfriend or your sister or your mother-in-law to join that yoga class with you. After all, exercise is good for their health too.

Furthermore, experts are sure that workouts go better for everyone if they're performed in teams. If you and your partner are lifting, you really need a spotter in order to safely push yourself. If you're playing a sport for fitness, like tennis, squash, or basketball, you'll need an opponent just to get a game going. And, in almost every fitness case, people are more likely to stick to their routines if they regularly perform them with a partner. It makes it more fun, which makes you

more likely to keep doing it. And it's harder to quit when you know you're letting down a partner.

And there's a bonus: It seems almost inevitable that working out with someone strengthens your relationship with her. Of course, your relationship will benefit from spending more time together—that's what got you in this mess in the first place. But the bond that is formed through mutual physical exhaustion is strangely perpetual, just ask the nation's frat boys about their pledge activities. You might find a new appreciation for your lover's body, your best friend's determination, or your father's strength when you begin to train with them. And they'll develop a similar regard for you.

The truth is that fitness is probably not more important than your job and your family. But, the truth is also that exercise is really quite good for you. That's why you got into it in the first place, and why you have the right to declare it as a priority at all. If you can get your job or your loved ones to agree with you, then you've got the perfect setup. If they're not there yet, then the challenge is to balance your time so that it reflects your priorities.

As long as you don't get carried away, then it's natural for those who care about you to respect and even appreciate your commitment to your health.

10
OBLIQUE
OBSESSION

A nyone who has ever enjoyed the heady endorphin rush after a great workout knows that becoming obsessed with exercise and fitness is only a health club membership (or a subscription to Men's Health) away. We've all seen the jogging junkie running at 6 a.m. in the rain or the fitness freak rushing off to the gym even though he's got pneumonia and two broken legs. Like a drug, fitness is addictive and the more one does it, the more addicted one is likely to get. (What do you think happened to Jack LaLanne? And it wasn't just by wearing those ridiculous jumpsuits!)

However, just like anything else, too much of a good thing isn't always so good. Shin splints, bone spurs, pulled hamstrings, multiple divorces, and even unemployment can all be the result of an exercise program gone horribly, terribly wrong.

What can you do to avoid a blistering case of "oblique obsession?" Read this chapter, for starters.

FEEL THE (AFTER)BURN

Being healthy and fit in the new millennium requires consistent training, daily motivational pep talks, and, of course, weekly massages. If you're on the fast track to fitness, you're eating right and working out on a daily basis. You're lean, you're buff, and you tend to piss everyone off because you're so healthy and energetic. But, like everything in life, things sometimes happen to

throw you off track. Anything from pregnancy to having the mother-in-law visit is cause for the usual workout program to go right out the window. Life's little interventions are no reason for you to put exercise on hold, however. So, if you're looking for excuses to skip your workout, you're out of luck.

Sports to SPICE UP your EXERCISE ROUTINE

- Tennis
- Soccer
- Hockey
- Basketball
- Boxing
- Racquetball
- Softball
- Golf
- Mountain/road biking
- Swimming

HITTING THE WALL (DON'T BONK)

Everyone hits the wall at some point in their fitness lives. This is called "bonking," and it happens to even the most committed fitness fiend. Bonking usually occurs when you've reached your limit. It may be emotional (your girlfriend could test the patience of a saint) or it may be physical (that last load of laundry *really* did you in), but either way, your body just refuses to go on any longer.

When your body rebels against all activity, you may be tempted to crawl into bed and forego life on the outside altogether. While throwing yourself a pity party can be fun, it's not the best solution. When you're emotionally or physically drained, the best thing you can do is to get up and move around no matter how crappy you feel. Maybe you can't handle your usual weekly basketball game or four-mile jog, and that's fine. This is a great opportunity to explore a less strenuous task, like yoga or a leisurely walk around the block. Doing anything physical will help you keep your energy up, which is just what you need to deal with life's petty little problems.

An illness is a different matter. When you're sick, your body is really busy feeling like crap and it's probably telling you to get in bed and stay there for the duration. If you've got the flu or anything else that brings on fever or upper-respiratory infections, bed rest is probably a good idea. You know to drink plenty of fluids, sleep a lot, and whine until your significant other murders you in your sleep. But what about exercise? Is it okay to keep exercising when you're sick? If you've got a little cold, you're fine (really, get out of bed and stop your bellyaching). Just tone it down and shorten your workouts a little.

Most illnesses are fairly benign and you can usually do the minimum amount of exercise (three times a week for 30 minutes) without losing all that endurance and muscle you've been working on. If you're recovering from a long illness that has left you weak and flabby, getting back into the usual routine will take time.

Unfortunately, it doesn't take long for your heart to forget all that great kick boxing or running you did for the last six months, so you have to remind it by slowly introducing it to light exercise. You might consider swimming or walking, since both are easy on the body and you can go as slowly as you want. Give yourself rest days in between your workouts and eat lots of gooey chocolate things to make yourself feel better. (Food is love, no?)

TO LIFT OR NOT TO LIFT

If you've been sick for a while, your usual weight lifting routine isn't going to do. Your body is weak and it can barely get out of bed right now, much less lift something repeatedly. Still, something is better than nothing, so instead of ignoring your dumbbells altogether, pick up some really light ones and work your major muscle groups.

To keep your muscles in the swing of things, simply do one exercise for each muscle (chest, back, shoulders, biceps, triceps, abs, and legs). Do one set for each exercise and then call it a day. This will at least

maintain the muscle you've built up until now and your bedsores will thank you for getting up! If you can manage this once or twice a week until you're fully recovered, getting back to your usual 50 pushups won't be quite as hard, although it will still be a bitch.

BURNOUT

Ah, the dreaded burnout. It happens to almost everyone who plays a sport or exercises on a regular basis. Total burnout means a daily feeling of dread when thinking of any kind of exercise. When you wake up in the morning and the thought of putting on your running shoes makes you want to stab yourself in the eye with a fork, that's a clue that your mind thinks your body is tired of your morning runs. Burnout is a hard obstacle to overcome because it lives in your mind rather than in your body. Mind over matter is a nice little cliché, but it's never easy to convince your mind of something it's dead set against.

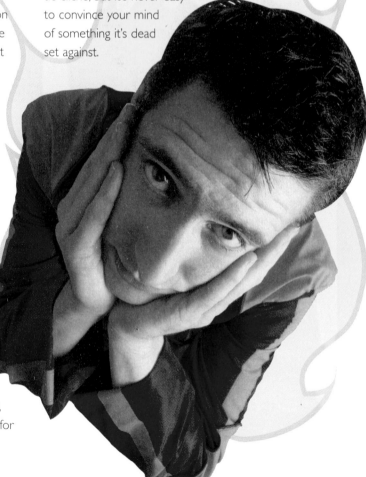

(Otherwise, we'd all visit our mother-in-laws daily.)

What your little brain is telling you is that it doesn't want to do the usual routine. It craves something new, unusual, and fun. Instead of taking a few months off from exercise altogether, why not completely change your routine so that it doesn't even resemble a normal day for you? If you usually work out at the gym, find somewhere else to exercise. Go get a set of dumbbells and lift weights while you're watching TV. Instead of always doing aerobics or kick boxing, get outside and walk or start a running program. Get a workout video or take a belly dancing class. The point is to be creative. The only requirement for exercise is that you raise your heart rate for 30 minutes or more and this can easily be done with anything from sex to cutting the grass.

BACK IN THE SADDLE

The most important thing you can do when getting your body back in line is to take your time. You've been exercising for a while, so you know your body and you know when you've gone too far. You can't expect to be down with the flu for three weeks and then skip out the door for a speed walking session. Instead, you may find yourself huffing and puffing by the time you reach the mailbox. This is a great time for a pep talk but, if you're all out of pep, just remind yourself that it may take a couple of weeks to get back to where you were. This is also a great time to baby yourself and to demand that others do the same.

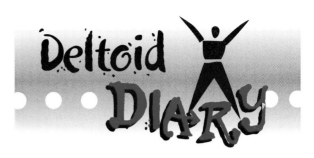

Deltoid Diary

I Love (Running in) New York

I woke up feeling awful. Seven gin and tonics. "Cassie," I mumbled. Nothing. I turned on the television. On Channel 2, they were broadcasting the New York City Marathon, which ended steps away from us in Central Park.

"Cassie," I said, hoping my roommate would hear my call. "I want to go watch the finish."

She thought I was crazy. "Who wants to run 26 miles? Who wants to run one mile?" she said. But we find ourselves, later, in the park. Cassie practically cursing the front-runners in disgust. "Are you people insane?" she cried. I stood next to her, transfixed. "This is beautiful," I said. "I'm going to do this next year." Did I believe myself? I wasn't sure. But I found myself thinking about it more and more, and then I found myself lining up in Central Park months later on a chilly April morning to get my application. It was a whimsical, spur of the moment decision made together with a boy I barely knew. I hadn't even been running with him yet; I wasn't even sure if he *could* run. He asked me, in line, "So, when was the last time you went running?"

"Yesterday," I said. "I ran around the park. I run all the time." His face turned a little pale. Apparently, I was more prepared than I thought. He ended up dropping out before training even started.

Training for something like this in New York City does not have the suburban amenities (winding country roads, silence, the crunch of leaves below one's feet) that made me fall in love with running. Three times around Central Park to complete the weekend's workout was utter drudgery. Especially if you had a particularly nauseating techno song that you'd picked up in a deli stuck in your head for the entire three hours and obnoxious inline skaters taking up half the roadway.

In the park, you also risked being trampled by horse-drawn carriages or being swept up in some kind of haphazard charity bike race. Of course, the other running alternative was Sixth Avenue, which, I found out, had a street fair nearly every weekend of the summer. Unless you woke up at 7 a.m., you were bombarded by slow-walking, camera waving pedestrians who curiously tried to photograph your pain. Not to mention that the smell of Italian sausage was not the most enticing odor after you've already sweated through 12 miles.

My health choices during training were not to be admired. My lunches often consisted of ice cream and Tootsie Rolls. I could eat anything. One night before running 20 miles I had a gourmet meal of cheese. I liked cheese so much that I didn't feel like making the lifestyle change to cut it out of my diet, 26 miles facing me or not. Nor did I ever stretch; it bored me. Why waste the time pulling on one's legs and arms? I'd rather be running and then deal with it later.

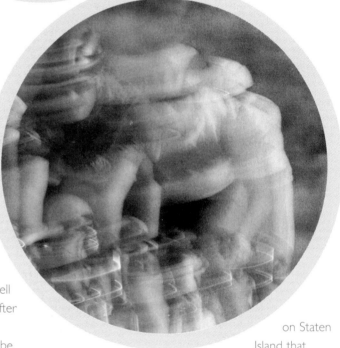

The morning of the race I climbed onto our marathon shuttle bus along with other people similarly overbundled in fleece, mittens, and sweaters. It was 6 a.m. and freezing. The woman next to me looked nervous. "I was talked into doing this by my friends," she admitted. "I've only run three times since September, and it's November 7th!" She then took a healthy bite out of her bagel and shrugged. "Whatever. I just hope I don't pee in my pants."

We were shuttle-bussed to a little army camp on Staten Island that overlooks the Verrazano Bridge (which is the starting point of the race). Inside the camp, there was a large inflatable Gatorade bottle; people swarmed around it and emerged from it swaddled in large, bright yellow garbage bags with the words GATORADE plastered all over them. Was this supposed to emit warmth? There was nowhere to go indoors; instead we were expected to huddle outside.

We had the option of sitting underneath tents. People snuggled very close to the ground, apparently in hopes of gathering heat from the soil.

It was very quiet except for the angry mob by the bagel table; apparently they'd run out of Nutella spread. With the vast European contingency of participants, a shortage of Nutella was a severe emergency. Luckily, reinforcements arrived, and the crowd swarmed to the bagels again, their faces soon awash in chocolate hazelnut goo. Napkins, at this point, were being salvaged for toilet paper.

The women lined up to start in front of the men. Several men jumped in our line to get a faster start; they were discovered and promptly ejected. Suddenly, I had to pee. Someone beside me said, "Just go more into the middle of the crowd and do it, no one will care." Afterwards I felt much better, although I think I ruined someone's shoes.

The start was announced by a cannon. No one expected it to go off, and when it did, this woman behind me shoved me so hard I was certain she was a man. I turned around in annoyance to see this excited, weathered little face. "Hello!" she waved a mitten at me. I wondered if she'd peed her pants.

I don't recall very much during the actual race. At every mile volunteers offered the runners cups of Gatorade or water. I'd slapped a Breathe Right strip on my nose, but after its Gatorade bath, the Breathe Right promptly fell off. I needed the water to wash off my hands as they gathered Gatorade stickiness, almost more than I needed it to drink. The wind became irrelevant after a while, and some of the neighborhoods were stark and beautifully quiet. The louder neighborhoods were host to country rock bands and testy spectators who would pummel you if you stopped to tie your shoe. "Keep running!" They'd scream. "Why are you stopping?"

On the Queensboro Bridge I wondered in desperation how much longer I would have to run uphill. Swept down from it, finally, I shot on to First Avenue, which was yet another hill. But it was fantastically empty, devoid of cars but full of people hauling themselves toward the Bronx, 16 miles in, wondering where they'd find the strength for the last 10.

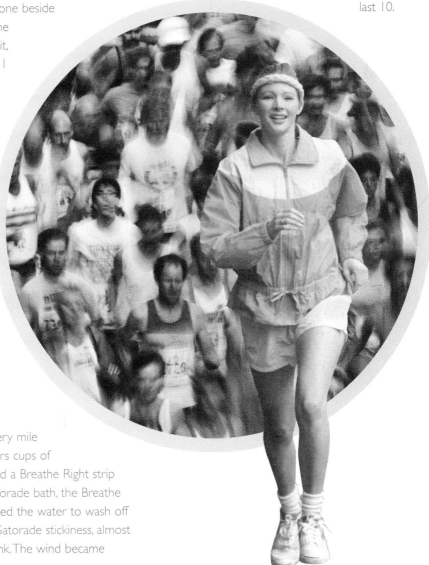

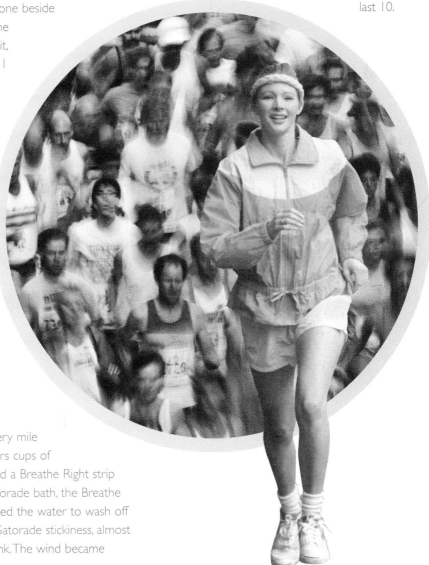

Somewhere in the Bronx a kid passed me a Nestlé Crunch. I gobbled it up and immediately thought I was going to vomit. The kid was probably laughing behind me. God I hated this city.

The second-to-last turn was onto 59th street and Central Park South. At this point I didn't feel particularly human. Furthermore, I was confused and thought we were on Central Park West and suddenly lost my mind. I forgot my name. I forgot what the hell I was doing. So I walked for a minute. My will came back, slowly, and I sputtered to finish. I hadn't lost my mind, I hadn't lost my legs, and, when I found my near-frozen cheering section, I ate a proffered black and white cookie, straight from some old-school deli, no doubt, in about a half a bite.

Despite the obstacles, running in New York is simply wonderful.

BACK ON
(THE NORDIC) TRACK

You rolled off the diet wagon and bounced over to the nearest donut hut. The cobwebs on your jogging shorts are so thick they look like lace. But, that's okay, because you can't fit into them anymore anyway. Had enough?

Good, because that kind of thinking has no place in an exercise program. People are not perfect. Setbacks are going to happen in an exercise program. The important thing is not to let your perceived failures crush your spirit. Take it for what it is, a learning experience, and move on to be stronger for it.

The fall, bounce, and/or roll from the exercise wagon can be traumatic. You wake up surrounded by candy wrappers and soda cans, or you stagger into your kitchen tripping over take-out taco wrappers and pizza boxes. You realize that you can once again feel your butt against the backs of your legs. Once the horror has passed, the thing to do is let it go and forgive yourself. Although it is important to track your program overall, it is best to approach its execution on a one-day-at-a-time basis. Yesterday is gone and there is nothing you can do to change it. Think of the past as one more thing in your "out box."

Similarly, do not fret about the future. Do not think of all the work you must do in order to catch up. Focus only on the task at hand, which is today's exercise. Someone said, "Right actions for the future are the best

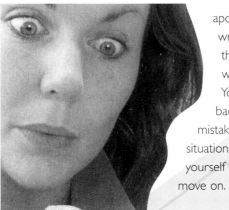

apologies for wrong ones in the past." He was right.

You cannot go back and undo mistakes or redo situations. So, give yourself a break and move on. Here's how.

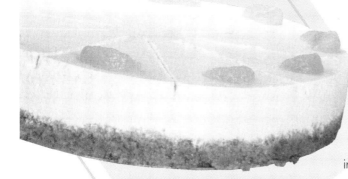

TRICEPS tip

Maintain your course.
If you fall off your routine for a time because of injury or illness, just get right back on when you feel better. Interruptions are part of life, don't let them make yours any harder.

Aerobic Analysis

In order to get on track, it is imperative to analyze what went wrong. Whether you went banana-nut bread nuts in the bakery section of your grocery store or you were forcefully asked to leave the corner buffet ("You no come back!"), you need to determine what triggered your binge. There are several common triggers for binge eating. These include starving yourself, getting emotional, gorging at festive occasions, and using a food reward system. The key to getting back on track is to figure out what triggered your binge eating and how to avoid a recurrence.

No Skipping!

It is very tempting to skip meals when dieting. This is one of the worst things you can do. It has a number of ill effects on your body. Your body needs fuel to

work properly. When you do not eat enough, your body will begin to feed on itself in order to survive. You will not lose fat. You will lose muscle. In fact, your body will store fat, as it prepares for a period of starvation. Because your body is burning muscle, you will lose muscle mass and tone. Further, you will experience headaches and stomachaches, irritability, loss of concentration, and lack of energy. All of these things will pave the road to binge eating.

When you get hungry, your resistance is down. It is much more difficult to control what you eat, how much you eat, and how quickly you eat. You will not be craving the light chicken breast and side salad. You will want the double cheeseburger and chili cheese fries. You also will not chew each bite

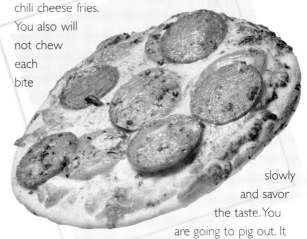

slowly and savor the taste. You are going to pig out. It takes 20 minutes for your body to register being full. If you eat slowly, you often find that you are full before you have eaten your entire meal. However, when you are pigging out, you will be amazed just how much you can get down your throat in that same 20 minutes. You will probably end up with a stomachache. However, this time it will be because you have eaten way too much.

Emotional Triggers

Emotional swings can trigger hunger. Being angry, lonely, tired, or depressed can push even the staunchest person into an eating binge. All of these emotions lead to the "What the &#@$" attitude. When you feel upset, food can be very comforting. When we were children, we were often given treats to make us feel better or to reward us for doing something special. Warm memories often revolve around sharing a meal or a dessert. High caloric memories of holidays, birthdays, and Sunday dinners can bring comforting feelings to us when we feel vulnerable or upset.

However, food offers only temporary comfort. Often, they lead to deeper feelings of depression, remorse, and guilt. It is better to find another way to deal with these emotions. Try meditation, talking with a friend, a warm bath, or even a good night's sleep. The trick is to deal with your emotions with your mind and not your mouth.

Happiness is also an emotional trigger. People often feel that it is okay to splurge while in a festive atmosphere. This is especially true when alcohol is involved. Summertime and the holidays are especially difficult for watching what you eat. There are so many tasty and fattening things all over the place. You can do several things to help yourself in this situation.

For instance, eat before you go. If you do not have an empty stomach, you will be less likely to pig out. Also, watch your alcohol intake. Drinking alcohol lowers your inhibitions and your resolve to watch what you are eating. Use the buddy system. You will be less likely to binge if someone is watching and supporting you. Finally, have water with you at all times, and drink it often to keep you full.

Reward!

Never use food as a reward! Further, be careful when thinking, "I have done so well, I deserve this entire cake." A treat here and there is fine. However, you should never feel entitled to splurge or binge because you have done well on your program. Instead of food, treat yourself to a massage, a new outfit, or a new toy. Yep, trade binge eating for binge shopping. It is very motivating to treat yourself to something related to your fitness program. New shoes, clothes, or pieces of equipment will help keep you focused on your program while also being a reward. Food is nourishment. Food is not a hobby or a reward.

Slim Scheduling

Poor scheduling refers to the times you have set for yourself to exercise. It is important to exercise at a time of day you feel energized. If you are a morning person, you should exercise in the morning. If you schedule your workouts for a time of day when you are usually drained, you are setting yourself up for failure. Although exercising will invigorate you, it takes a tremendous amount of discipline and dedication to get started when you are tired. You may have this type of discipline and dedication on any given day, but it is asking a lot to do this every day. Exercise will become just another chore you do not really want to do. If it is not fun, and it is not required, you will not do it for very long. Be creative. Try breaking up your workouts. Walk for 30 minutes at lunch, and then do your weight training after work. As long as you do the aerobics in blocks of at least 15 to 30 minutes, you will be fine. If you hate your exercise, change it. Figure out what it is about the exercise that does not agree with you, and choose something else.

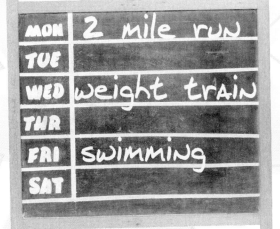

MON	2 mile run
TUE	
WED	weight train
THR	
FRI	swimming
SAT	

Holly Daze

It is easy to get sidetracked by holidays, vacations, traveling, and illness. The thing is, there will always be something. You have to decide what is important and go from there. If you are traveling for business or pleasure, there are still things you can do. Often, hotels offer gym facilities or a pool. Even if you cannot do your regular routine, do what you can. For instance, you can do push-ups, sit-ups, squats, lunges, etc., in any room. If weather and scenery permit, go for a walk or a jog. The same idea holds true for the holiday season. When your schedule does not seem like your own anymore, squeeze in what you can when you can.

Sick vs. Sweat?

Finally, if you have been ill or injured, the important thing is to get healthy. Pushing yourself when you are not well or if you are injured will only prolong your condition. If you have an injury to a part of your body that does not hinder you exercising the other parts, do that. For instance, if you break your foot, ask your doctor if it is okay for you to work out doing sitting upper body weight training. Once you are back to 100 percent, hit your program with renewed enthusiasm and appreciation for your health.

Fitness Forgiveness

Regardless of why you fell out of sync with your exercise program, the important thing is to forgive yourself and start again. Figure out what happened. Analyze your food triggers. Re-evaluate and adjust your program. It is not the end of the world to fail; it is the end of the world to quit. So, no matter how many times you fall, bounce, roll, or jump off that wagon, just make sure you get back on with all the lessons you have learned.

WEEKEND WARRIORS

When physical activity during the work week consists of power walking from your desk to the coffee pot so you can fill your cup before the coffee disappears or jumping up and madly sprinting to the conference room to solve the next company crisis, you have to be careful not to overdo the exercising on the weekends. Trying to make up for lost activity during the week by power exercising on the weekends can be dangerous. How many of us have felt like slugs after sitting in a cubicle all week, so we try to make up for it by getting in shape in one weekend? We pretend to be Superman on Saturday, only to find that on Sunday we don't have the strength of Mighty Mouse to roll out of bed.

Does this scenario sound familiar? Saturday morning you jump out of bed, throw on the running shoes, and jog to the gym to meet your personal trainer. The trainer puts you through an intensive weight workout, three sets of endurance lifts followed by three sets of strengthening lifts. However, you decide that because you've felt like a slug all week maybe you should do the whole workout one more time after the trainer leaves.

After weight training you go to play some racquetball. Since you've spent all this money on a membership at the gym, (which you have only used twice in the last three months) you figure you are going to get your money's worth today while you are here, so after racquetball you take a step aerobics class.

Now you're beginning to feel a little tired. You figure you'll just go to that one late-afternoon yoga class to stretch out before you call it a day. After the opening meditation, however, the instructor announces that it's "power yoga" day. Uh-oh! By the time you finish, your legs feel like Jell-O, your back aches, and your arms shake when you try to lift them to open your locker. Putting on your shirt becomes a world-class effort. You think you, just maybe, might have overdone it.

You drag your shaky body out of the gym ready to get in your car and go home for a hot bath and a cold beer. In the fading twilight, you look for your car in the practically empty parking lot. That's when you realize, "Oh, yeah, I was Superman today. I ran."

By the time you finally struggle home, crawling part of the way, the bath and the beer are but distant memories. All you can think of is bed! You fall against the door as Sparky brings you his leash and asks you to take him for a walk. Sparky hasn't been out in days and you know how much he needs a walk, but you just can't muster the energy. Pushing him aside, you struggle to your room and collapse into bed—without stretching. By the time Sunday rolls around, your plans for another tough workout day are shot. Your body feels like you've gone 10 rounds with Mike Tyson (yes, your ears hurt, too), and you worry that you might need a neck brace to get out of bed. Now you really feel like a slug, because one day of working out has turned you into a sniveling, crying, aching lump.

This entire scenario could have been easily avoided with a little planning and forethought. The idea that you can sit in a cubicle all week and then spend six hours in the gym on Saturday and still actually get out of bed and walk on Sunday is a pipe dream. In order to stay healthy year round, regular exercise is required. And that doesn't mean "regularly" sprinting to the break room to fill your coffee mug.

It is important to get some exercise during the week, even if it's not much. By keeping reasonably active during the week, you won't be starting at square one every Saturday. The human body begins to break down muscle and convert it to a better storage medium, fat, in as little as 36 hours if not properly maintained. By working out only on weekends, you lose any progress you may have made during the week while you're inactive. Some ways to keep your blood pumping during the week so that the weekend doesn't kill you are: taking the stairs in your home or office, walking to lunch, biking to work, and yes, even taking poor Sparky for a walk. If your house has stairs, instead of throwing the dirty laundry over the railing, or just dropping that book or letter to your sweetie down below, walk them down. At work, take the stairs up to your office rather than the elevator. Often, you can find a way to take the stairs when you visit the doctor's office or other professional buildings. Sometimes you have to look for the stairwell in places where the elevator is made more easily accessible. It is worth the search.

When you leave for lunch, pick a restaurant a few blocks away and walk there. Dodging midday traffic can be a good workout. Remember to keep it at a brisk walk. Stopping to chat with the newspaper vendor and buying a Snickers bar doesn't do any good.

Commuting to work by bicycle is not only a good way to squeeze a workout into the weekdays, but it's relaxing and invigorating to boot. Studies have shown that people who exercise before work—by either jogging or riding their bike to work—are more productive, less stressed, and generally happier than those who do not. This is easily understandable. Car commuters have been sitting in gridlock, dealing with traffic lights, and spilling their breakfast on their nice clean suit for the same 45 minutes that it has taken you to get there by bike.

An added benefit to riding your bike to work is convenient parking. While everyone else is muscling for that last spot in the lot, which is still a 5-minute walk to the building, or paying $10 to park, you can waltz right up to the door and lock your bike to the stairwell, or better yet, to the bumper of your boss' car sitting in that "reserved" spot. You could also get a great

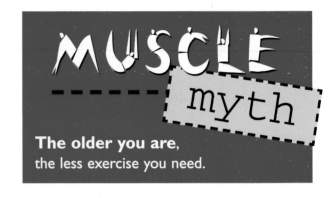

workout for your arms by carrying it up the stairs with you to your office and putting it in the corner for the day.

Sure, you might get just a little sweaty, but that's only because you don't do it all the time, yet. After a while, your metabolism will boost, and taking the stairs or riding your bike to work won't even get your heart rate up. If you really are concerned about your post-stairwell stench causing your neighbors' eyes to water and their hair to shrivel up and fall out, you can change clothes at the office. Bring the suit and tie with you, or keep a spare change of clothes at work. You can use a damp washcloth or baby towelettes under your arms to keep the aroma down.

The other key to avoiding the Saturday full-workout action turning into the Sunday full-body

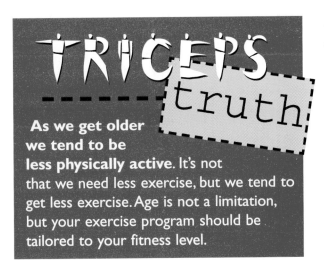

TRICEPS truth

As we get older we tend to be less physically active. It's not that we need less exercise, but we tend to get less exercise. Age is not a limitation, but your exercise program should be tailored to your fitness level.

traction is pacing. Moderation is the key to good health, whether it be in food, drink, sleep, or fitness. By listening to your body and being careful to only push it as far as it's capable, you can enjoy activity all weekend without having it hurt you. Also, remember to take care of yourself by eating right and properly warming up and cooling down. An important aspect of exercising is stretching. Stretch before and after every workout.

Start out Saturday morning with a nutritious breakfast. You'll want to eat something that is light, but fortifying. Try some fruit or cereal. After breakfast, take the time to stretch out. But, don't stretch too hard! The best time to stretch is when your muscles are warm. You need to loosen your muscles up first, so do some easy stretching followed by something that warms up the body.

For example, rather than running to the gym, try a brisk walk. That way you can warm up without overdoing it. Once you get to the gym, then do your deep stretching routine there. When the trainer puts you through your workout, remember it or write it down to do again tomorrow, rather than doing it again right away.

Snacking throughout the day is a good idea, too. Bring apples or vegetable sticks to munch on as you go. Your body will do better and you'll have a more effective workout if you give it the vitamins and carbohydrates it needs to keep going. Besides, this will keep you from going to Taco Bell after your workout because you're too hungry to make it home. Drink lots of water to flush the lactic acid buildup from your tissue. This lactic acid is one of the biggest causes of muscle fatigue. Water helps reduce this buildup so you can work out longer and will be less sore the next day.

Keep stretching throughout the day. Stretch, stretch, stretch. That way when you show up to the yoga class, you won't hurt yourself because you'll already be stretched out.

Perhaps the biggest key to working out on the weekends if you don't work out during the week is this: Don't be too hard on yourself. You don't have to knock yourself out because you haven't done anything during the week. Think positively about the fact you are going to work out now.

If you still feel like running home after a light to moderate day at the gym, go for it. If you've been taking care of yourself all day, stretching and trying to maintain at least a minimum activity level during the week, you can probably do it and still lift your head off the pillow in the morning. When you get home make a healthy dinner. Eating right makes working out that much more rewarding. Or, if you're too tired, you can always go to that all-you-can-eat salad buffet.

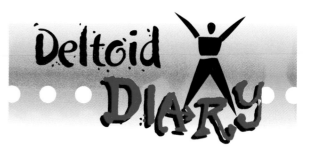

Deltoid DIARY

The Perfumed Bandit

Certain oddities seem to gravitate toward certain places and venues. No one knows why such instances occur where and when they do, but only that it has become a reality. Such is the case when exploring the parameters of the health-conscious world. The local gym is a breeding ground for a curiosity that can only be described as the "Perfumed Bandit." This character can be defined as the woman found positioned at various locales in a busy gym but who is not partaking in any aerobic or anaerobic activity.

For some reason, she looks out of place, because her appearance leads a person to believe that she is at some other event, rather than a place for sweaty and out of breath clientele. She doesn't acknowledge the fact that her outward appearance is not in keeping with the norm, and her attitude doesn't reflect a need for change. And she doesn't appear to be alone. No. So that one is better equipped to handle such a person when presented with the opportunity, an explanation of the offending image is definitely in order.

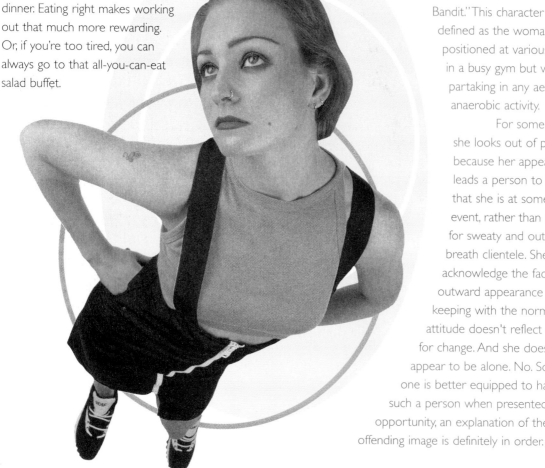

To begin, let us look at the label. The latter word, Bandit, refers to the time they steal away from seemingly disciplined exercisers, as they lounge on equipment, surveying the area for possible conversationalists. Seemingly unbeknownst to them is the fact that their fellow gym goers seek the refuge of the equipment to further enhance their figures or health status. As the fearless soldiers strive on toward attaining fulfillment, these creatures continuously plot to foil them, by wreaking havoc on their exercise routines. Gotta use the bench? Too bad, some chick's handbag has taken up residence there. Oh, and the owner of the object in question? Trying to lure away the overpumped muscle-bound guy on the machine to your left. Seems like a losing battle, as the guy has fallen victim to her overly made-up lashes and caked-on eye shadow. And butting into the conversation at this point would not be recommended. Not if you value your health, anyway.

Now let us explore the first half of the expression, "Perfumed." Although this aspect seems quite self-explanatory, there is still room to educate the unaware. This is a violation of the olfactory senses, as anyone with common knowledge knows the death of a good, invigorating workout is breathing in excessive fumes from a woman's perfume.

Please note though, for the sake of equality, that men can also be accused of bathing in way too much cologne prior to hitting the gym.

So with a solid preface to the creature at hand, please be aware of this image when next frequenting a health club. You now have the information to visually assess the "Perfumed Bandit" upon initial contact, and if in doubt, can definitely remind your sense of smell where the offender originates from.

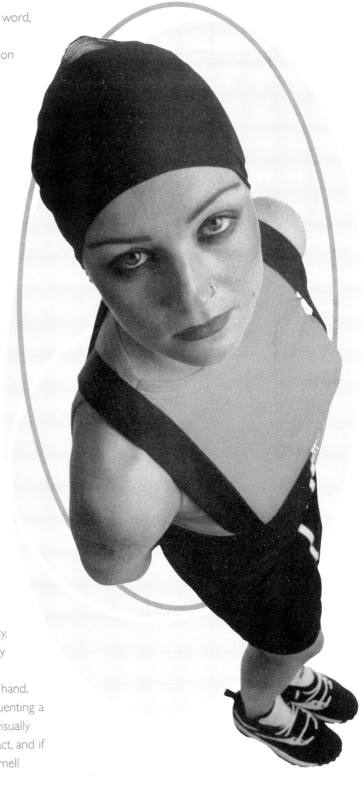

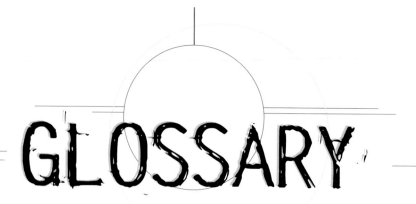

GLOSSARY

Like any specialized pursuits, exercising and fitness training have a language all their own. The following is a glossary of the most commonly used terms you might hear being tossed around at the gym.

A

Abdominals
The collective name for the muscles on the front of the torso, below the chest.

Abduction
The movement of a limb away from the middle of the body, such as bringing your arms to shoulder height from a hanging down position.

"Abs"
Abbreviation for abdominal muscles.

Absolute Strength
The maximum amount a person can lift in one repetition.

Accommodating Resistance
Increasing the resistance as a lifter's force increases through range of motion. Nautilus machines are said to provide accommodating resistance.

Acquired Aging
The acquisition of characteristics commonly associated with aging but that are actually caused by immobility or sedentary living.

Active Stretch
Muscles are stretched using the contraction of the opposing muscle. For example, stretching the triceps requires the biceps to contract.

Adduction
Movement of a limb toward the middle of the body, such as bringing your arms to the side from an extended position at the shoulder.

Adductors
Muscles of the inner thigh that pull your legs together. They attach the pelvis and the femur (or thigh bone).

Adenosine Diphosphate (ADP)
ADP is formed when ATP (adenosine triphosphate) is broken down within the body's

cell furnace, otherwise known as the mitochondria. This provides energy for muscular contraction.

Adhesion
Fibrous patch holding muscles or other parts together that are normally separated.

Aerobic
A low-intensity, sustained activity that relies on oxygen for energy. Aerobic activity builds endurance, burns fat, and conditions the cardiovascular system. To attain an aerobic effect you must increase your heart rate to 65 to 85 percent of your maximum heart rate, and maintain this level for at least 20 minutes. Examples of aerobic exercise include running, brisk walking, bicycling, and swimming.

Aerobic Capacity
Another term for maximal oxygen uptake (VO2 Max).

Agonist
A muscle directly engaged in contraction that is primarily responsible for movement of a body part.

Aikido
A Japanese martial art.

"All Natural"
Popular term for athletes, especially bodybuilders, who can avoid using steroids or other banned substances.

All-or-None
An exercise in which muscle fiber contracts fully or it does not contract at all.

American Federation of Women Bodybuilders (AFWB)
The group that oversees women's amateur bodybuilding in America.

American Physique Committee, Inc. (APC)
The group that oversees men's amateur bodybuilding in America.

Amino Acids
The twenty-two basic building blocks of the body that make up proteins.

Anabolic Steroid
A synthetic chemical that mimics the muscle-building characteristics of the male hormone testosterone.

Anaerobic Exercise
High-intensity exercise that burns glycogen for energy instead of oxygen. Anaerobic exercise creates a temporary oxygen debt by consuming more oxygen than the body can supply. An example of anaerobic exercise includes weightlifting.

Anaerobic Threshold
The point at which you begin working your muscles without oxygen, from an aerobic level, believed to be at about 87% of your maximum heart rate.

Angina Pectoris
Chest or arm pain resulting from reduced oxygen supply to the heart muscle.

Antagonist
A muscle that counteracts the agonist by lengthening when the agonist muscle contracts.

Anti-Catabolism
Supplements such as glutamine, used to prevent breakdown within the body, in order to promote muscle growth.

Antioxidants
Substances such as Vitamins A, C, and E and minerals such as copper, magnesium, and zinc. Believed to destroy free radicals, which some scientists believe may not only accelerate aging but also contribute to the formation of cancers and cataracts.

Arm Blaster
Aluminum or fiberglass strip supported at waist height by a strap around the neck. Keeps elbows from moving while curling barbells or dumbbells or doing triceps pushdowns.

Aromatherapy
Therapy incorporating the use of fragrant, natural, botanical essential oils from plants, leaves, bark, roots, seeds, resins, and flowers.

Arteriosclerosis
Hardening of the arteries due to conditions that cause the arterial walls to become thick, hard, and non-elastic.

Asana
The proper term for any of the many poses performed in yoga.

Assimilation
The process in which foods are utilized and absorbed by the body.

Atherosclerosis
The depositing of materials along the arterial walls, a type of arteriosclerosis.

Atrophy
Decrease in size and functional ability of tissue or organs, such as the muscles.

B

"Baby's Butt"
Popular term for the indentation between the two heads of the biceps muscles of a very muscular athlete.

Back Cycling
Cutting back on either number of sets, repetitions, or amount of weight used during an exercise session.

Ballistic Stretch
A kind of stretching that advocates bouncing to increase the amount of stretch. This is no longer recommended as it has been found to cause muscle tears and soreness.

Bar
The metal rod that forms the handle of a barbell or dumbbell.

Barbell
A basic piece of equipment used in strength training. A barbell consists of a bar, sleeve, collars, and weights or plates. Barbells can be of a fixed weight or a variable weight.

Basal Metabolic Rate (BMR)
The number of calories consumed by the body while at rest. This is measured by the rate at which heat is given off, and is expressed in calories per hour per square meter of skin surface.

Bicep
The muscle running along the inside of the upper arm which bends your arm at the elbow.

Bioavailability
The rate at which nutrients can be absorbed.

Biochemical Reaction
The chemical reactions that take place within the human body.

Biological Value
A measure of protein quality in a given food.

Biomechanics
The science concerned with the internal and external forces acting on a human body and the effects produced by these forces.

Body Composition
The breakdown of your body makeup, such as fat, lean muscle, bone, and water content.

Body Composition Test
Computerized evaluation of lean body mass determining the percentage of body fat.

Body Fat
The percentage of your body mass that is not composed of lean muscle, water, bones, or vital organs.

Bodybuilding
Weight training to change your physical appearance.

Bone Density
Soundness of the bones within the body; low density can be a result of osteoporosis.

"Buffed"
Slang for good muscle size and definition.

Buffer
Substances that help reduce lactic acid buildup during strenuous exercise.

Bulking Up
Gaining body weight by adding muscle, body fat, or both.

Burn
The sensation in a muscle when it has been worked intensely. It is caused by fatigue by-products and microscopic muscle tears. In endurance exercise, working muscles until lactic acid build-up causes burning sensation. (As in "going for the burn.")

Burnout
State of being bored or tired with exercise, frequently the result of over-training or unvaried workouts. Cross-training and rest are good remedies for burnout.

C

Cadence
The beat, time, or measure of rhythmic motion or activity, such as pedaling a bicycle. Your "cadence" is the speed of your pedaling.

Carbohydrate Loading
Increased consumption of carbohydrates in liquid or food form, normally occurring three days prior to an endurance type of event.

Carbohydrates
Compounds that contain carbon, hydrogen, and oxygen used by the body as a fuel source. Two main groups are sugars and starch.

"Carbs"
Slang term for carbohydrates.

Cardiovascular
Relating to or involving the heart and blood vessels.

Cardiovascular Training
Physical conditioning that strengthens the heart and blood vessels, resulting in an increase in the ability of your body muscles to utilize fuel more effectively at a greater level of fitness.

Catabolism
The breakdown of lean muscles mass, normally as a result of injury, immobilization, and poor dieting techniques.

Cellulose
The indigestible fiber in foods.

Chalk
Powder used on the hands for a secure grip on exercise equipment, such as a weight bar.

Cheating
Too much weight used in an exercise, therefore relying on surrounding muscle groups for assistance in the movement; or changing joint angles for more leverage, as in arching your back in a bench press.

Cholesterol
A fat lipid which has both good and bad implications within the human body. "Good" being known as HDL and "bad" being LDL. Bad cholesterol is associated with heart disease and stroke, whereas the body requires good cholesterol for the production of many steroid hormones.

Circuit Weight Training
A routine that combines light to moderate-intensity weight training with aerobic training. A circuit routine typically consists of 5 to 10 stations set up at close intervals. The object is to move from station to station with little rest between exercises, until the entire circuit has been completed.

Clean
Lifting weight from the floor to your shoulder in one motion.

Clean and Jerk
An Olympic lift in which weight is raised from the floor to an overhead position in two movements.

Clean and Snatch
One of two Olympic lifts in which weight is raised from the floor to an overhead position at arms' length in one motion.

Coenzyme
A substance that works with an enzyme to promote the enzyme's activity.

Collar
The clamp that holds the weight plates in position on a bar. There are inner collars and outer collars.

Colon Therapy
A high colonic enema that cleanses using water. Benefits include detoxification, cleansing of the blood, and the stimulation of internal organs.

Complete Proteins
Proteins that contain all the essential amino acids.

Complex Carbohydrates
Starches, such as grains, breads, rice, pasta, vegetables, and beans. They get their name from

their complex, chainlike structure. During digestion, starches are typically broken down into sugars and used by the body for energy.

Compound Training
Sometimes called "giant sets": doing 3 to 4 exercises for the same muscle, one after the other, with little to no rest in between.

Compression Wrap
A localized treatment for cellulite and fatty deposits on arms, legs, and buttocks.

Concentric Contraction
An isotonic muscle contraction, where a muscle contracts or shortens.

Congestive Heart Failure
The inability of the heart muscle to pump blood at a life-sustaining rate.

Contouring
Deep toning of muscles using calisthenics.

Contraction
The shortening and lengthening of a muscle that occurs while performing an exercise.

Cool Down
The practice of slowing down at the end of a workout to allow your body temperature and heart rate to decrease gradually.

Coronary Circulation
Circulation of blood to the heart muscle associated with the blood carrying capacity of a specific vessel or development of collateral vessels (extra blood vessels).

Coronary Heart Disease (CHD)
Diseases of the heart muscle and the blood vessels that supply it with oxygen, where

symptoms such as heart attack could occur.

Coronary Occlusion
The blocking of the coronary blood vessels.

Creatine Phosphate
A protein-like substance manufactured by your muscles (but also found in some meats) that has been found to increase athletic performance and delay fatigue.

Cross-training
The practice of mixing different activities into your regular workout routine to avoid overuse injuries and to prevent boredom. Cycling, running, and swimming are three common activities used to cross-train different muscle groups.

Crunches
Abdominal exercises in the form of sit-ups done on the floor with your legs on a bench and your hands behind your neck.

Curl Bar
Chambered bar designed for a more comfortable grip and less forearm strain during weight curls.

Curved Last
A kind of shoe construction with a curved sole. This shape provides cushioning and promotes inward motion. Good for feet with rigid, high arches that underpronate.

"Cut Up"
The popular term for a body that carries very little fat and is highly muscled.

"Cutting Up"
Slang for reducing body fat and water retention to increase muscle definition.

Cybex
Patented exercise equipment used for isokinetic strength training.

D

Dancercise
Modified modern dance steps and movements designed to provide an aerobic workout.

Dead Lift
One of three power lifting events (the other two are squat and bench press). Weight is lifted off the floor to approximately waist height. The lifter must stand erect, with shoulders back.

Deep Muscle Massage
A type of massage that eliminates knots, locked up areas, and emotional blocks in the body due to prolonged stress. It includes various leverage techniques and kneading for a very firm massage.

Deficiency
A sub-optimal level of one or more nutrients, often resulting in poor health.

Definition
A term that describes a muscle that is highly developed, the shape of which is clearly visible: A "cut up" muscle.

Dehydration
The abnormal depletion of body fluids, easily detected by dark, concentrated urine. Prevented by drinking water or sports drinks before, during, and after exercise.

Delayed Onset Muscle Soreness (DOMS)
A condition that is often felt after exercise, especially lifting heavy weight or excessive running. Caused by the micro tears within your muscles as part of the body rebuilding phase.

Deltoids
The triangular, tri-part muscles that wrap around the tops of the shoulders. They allow you to raise your arms forward, backward, and out to the sides and also rotate them inward and outward.

"Delts"
Abbreviation for deltoids.

Dip Belt
A large, heavy belt worn around the hips with a chain at each end that can be attached to a barbell plate or dumbbell for additional resistance during certain exercises like dips.

Diuretic
A substance that aids the increase of urine excreted by the body.

Double (Split Training) Routine
Working out twice a day to allow for shorter, more intense workouts. Usually performed by more advanced bodybuilders in preparation for a contest.

Drying Out
Encouraging the loss of body fluids by limiting fluid intake, eliminating salt, sweating heavily, and/or using diuretics.

Dumbbell
A one-handed barbell. Dumbbells are shorter and generally of a lighter weight than barbells. Often used in pairs.

E

Easy Set
Exercise not even close to maximum effort, as in a warm-up.

Eccentric Contraction
The act in which a muscle lengthens while still maintaining tension.

Electrolytes
Minerals such as sodium, potassium, calcium, and magnesium that act to keep your nerves firing and muscles moving, especially during exercise. They are lost through sweating and can be replaced by drinking sports drinks.

Endogenous
Naturally occurring body productions.

Endorphins
Any of a group of proteins with potent analgesic properties that occur naturally in the brain. These are the brain chemicals that contribute to the "runner's high" or good feelings during and after exercise.

Endurance
The ability of a muscle to produce force continually over a period of time.

Enzyme
Helpful protein molecules which are responsible for a multitude of chemical reactions within the body.

Ergogenic
Something that can increase muscular work capacity.

Ergometer
Exercise machine designed for muscular contraction.

Essential Fatty Acids (EFAs)
Required by the body, however only obtainable from food sources, such as flaxseed oil and safflower oil.

Estrogen
The female sex hormone.

Exercise
In weight training, the individual movements performed during a routine. In general, the movements required to complete a workout or an activity done for the purpose of keeping fit and healthy.

Extension
Body part (e.g. hand, neck, trunk) going from a bent to a straight position, as in a leg extension.

External Obliques
The muscles running diagonally downward and inward from the lower ribs to the pelvis that allow you to bend forward and twist at the waist. These lie on top of the internal obliques.

F

Failure
Being unable to complete a movement because of fatigue.

Fartlek
Swedish word for "speed play," a type of loosely structured interval training for runners, cyclists, and in-line skaters. It combines high-intensity segments

with your regular training pace in order to build strength and speed.

Fascia
Fibrous connective tissue that covers, supports, and separates all muscles and muscle groups. It also unites skin with underlying tissue.

Fast Twitch
Refers to muscle cells that fire quickly and are utilized in anaerobic activities such as sprinting and power lifting.

Fat
Often referred to as lipids or triglycerides, one of the main food groups, containing nine calories per gram. Fat serves a variety of functions in the body, however a high percentage of body fat has been proven to be unhealthy.

Fatigue
Physical weariness resulting from exertion.

Fibrin
The substance that in combination with blood cells forms a blood clot.

Flex
To bend or decrease the angle of a joint or contract a muscle.

Flexibility
Range of movement in a joint or group of joints or the ability of a bone joint or muscle to stretch. Good flexibility refers to an advanced degree of limberness in the joints and muscles.

Flexion
Bending in contrast to extending.

Floatation
Suspension in tanks filled with sterile salt water regulated so that its temperature is precisely the same as your body temperature for a sense of buoyancy and weightlessness.

Flush
To cleanse a muscle by increasing the blood supply to it, thus removing toxins left in the muscle by exertion.

Forced Repetitions
Assistance from others to perform additional repetitions of an exercise when your muscles can no longer complete the movement on their own.

Free-Form Amino Acids
Structurally unlinked individual amino acids.

Free Radicals
Highly reactive molecules that possess unpaired electrons.

Free style Training
Training many body parts in one workout.

Free Weights
Weights not attached to a machine or driven by cables or chains. Barbells and dumbbells are examples of free weights.

Fructose
Often used as a sugar substitute for diabetics, because of its low glycemic index. A healthier option than normal sugar, since fructose comes from fruit.

Full Spectrum Amino Acids
A supplement that contains all of the essential amino acids.

G

G5
A form of hand massage designed to relax tense muscles.

Glucagon
A hormone responsible for the regulation of blood sugar levels.

Glucose
A sugar, the usual form in which carbohydrates are assimilated by the body.

"Gluteals"
Abbreviation for gluteus maximus, medius, and minimus, otherwise known as the buttocks muscles.

"Glutes"
Slang term for gluteus maximus, medius, and minimus.

Gluteus Maximus, Medius, and Minimus
The three muscles of the buttocks and hips that extend your thighs forward and to the side (abduction) and rotate your legs at the hips.

Glycemic Index (GI)
A measuring system to find the extent to which various foods raise the blood sugar level. The benchmark is white bread, which has a GI of 100. The higher the score, the greater the extents of blood sugar raise.

Glycogen
The principal form of carbohydrate energy (glucose) stored within the body's muscles and liver.

Growth Hormone
An anabolic hormone naturally released by the pituitary gland. It promotes muscle growth and the breakdown of body fat for energy, greatly reduced after the age of about twenty.

H

Hamstrings
The group of three muscles on the back of your thighs that runs from the lower part of the pelvis to just below the knees. They allow you to bend your knees and straighten your legs at the hips.

Hand Off
Assistance from others in getting a weight to the starting position for an exercise.

Hard Set
To perform a prescribed number of repetitions of an exercise using maximum effort.

Health and Wellness Promotion
Altering lifestyles and environmental factors with the intent of improving quality of life.

Hellerwork
Deep tissue bodywork, stress reduction, and movement reeducation.

Herbal Wrap
The body is wrapped in a cloth soaked in a herbal solution to eliminate impurities, detoxify the body, and induce relaxation.

Herbology
Therapeutic use of herbs in treatments and diet.

High Density Lipoprotein (HDL)
A blood substance that picks up cholesterol and helps remove it from the body; often called "good cholesterol."

Holistic Health
A philosophy of well-being that considers the physical, mental, and spiritual aspects of life as closely interconnected and balanced.

Homeopathy
Based on the principle that "like cures like," this form of medicine treats patients with natural substances that cause symptoms much like those manifested by the ailment, thus stimulating the body to heal itself.

Hormones
Regulators of various biological processes through their ability to control the action of enzymes. Made from proteins, such as insulin for blood sugar control, or cholesterol for testosterone control.

Hydrotherapy
Water used as a form of treatment by way of jet massages, showers, and baths.

Hyperkinetic Condition
A disease/illness or health condition caused by or contributed to by excessive exercise.

Hypertension
High blood pressure.

Hypertrophy
The increase in the size of a muscle as a result of high-intensity weight training.

Hypoglycemia
A common occurrence in diabetics, otherwise known as low blood sugar levels, resulting in anxiety, fatigue, and a number of other conditions including coma and death.

I

Illness
Symptoms that upset your health.

Incomplete Proteins
Proteins which are low in one or more of the essential amino acids.

Intensity
The amount of force—or energy—you expend during a workout.

Internal Obliques
The muscles that run upward and inward from the hip bones to the lower ribs, allowing you to rotate and bend at the waist. These are located underneath the external obliques.

International Federation of BodyBuilders (IFBB)
The IFFB, founded in 1946, is a group that oversees world-wide men's and women's amateur and professional bodybuilding.

Intervals
Speed workouts, usually run on a track, which typically consist of relatively short sprints interspersed with rest periods of slower running.

Interval Training
A combination of high energy exercise followed by a period of low intensity activity.

Isokinetic Exercise

Isotonic exercise in which there is accommodating resistance. Nautilus is a type of isokinetic machine, where the machine varies the amount of resistance being lifted to match the force curve developed by the muscle.

Isolation

In weight training, confining an exercise to one muscle or one part of a muscle.

Isometric Exercise

Muscular contraction where the muscle maintains a constant length and joints do not move. These exercises are usually performed against a wall or some other immovable object.

Isotonic Exercise

Muscular action in which there is a change in length of muscle and weight, keeping the tension constant. Lifting free weights is a classic isotonic exercise.

J

Jin Shin Do

The ancient art of harmonizing life energy within the body by placing fingertips over clothing on designated areas.

"Just Do It!"

The famous marketing phrase used by the sports manufacturer Nike.

K

Kickboard

A small foam board used for short sprints to develop leg power and speed when swimming. Held under the chest so that the arms are not involved in the swimming stroke.

Kilometer

A metric measurement used in athletic events. One K equals 0.62 miles.

Kinesiology

The study of muscles and their movements.

Knee Wraps

Elastic strips used to wrap the knees for better support when performing squats, dead lifts, etc.

L

Lactic Acid (Lactate)

A by-product of anaerobic (or high intensity) exercise that collects in the muscles and causes soreness, stiffness, and fatigue.

Latissimus Dorsi

The pair of fan-shaped muscles across your middle and lower back that attach the arms to the spine. They work to pull your arms down and back, and give you good posture when they are toned.

"Lats"

Abbreviation for latissimus dorsi, the large muscles of the back that move the arms downward, backward, and in internal rotation.

Lean Body Mass

Everything in the body except for fat, including bone, organs, skin, nails, and all body tissue including muscle. Approximately 50 to 60% of lean body mass is water.

Lifestyle
Individual patterns of your daily life.

Lift Off
Assistance from others in getting a weight to its proper starting position.

Ligament
A strong, fibrous band of connecting tissue that connects bone to bone.

Lipids
All fats and fatty acids.

Lipoprotein
A fat-carrying protein in the blood.

Liposuction
The cosmetic procedure in which fat cells are surgically removed by a trained medical professional.

Lock Out
The partial repetition of an exercise by pushing the weight through only the last few inches of movement.

Low Density Lipoprotein (LDL)
A core of cholesterol surrounded by protein, often referred to as "bad cholesterol."

"Lower Abs"
Abbreviation for the abdominal muscles below the navel.

Low Impact Aerobics
A form of aerobics, minus the jumping, which spares the body possible injuries.

Lumbar
Lower region of your spine, also known as vertebrates L1 to L5. Used for bending and extending the body forward and backward, with the aid of the abdominal and erector spinae muscles.

M

Massage
The type of therapy based on the concepts of human function, anatomy, and physiology that uses a wide variety of soft tissue and manipulative techniques.

"Max"
Slang term for the maximum effort used for one repetition of an exercise.

Maximum Heart Rate
The fastest rate at which your heart should beat during exercise. To find your maximum rate, subtract your age from 220.

Midsection
The muscles of the abdominal area, including the upper and lower abdominals, obliques, and rectus abdominis muscles.

Military Press
Pressing a barbell from the upper chest upward in a standing or sitting position.

Mud Treatment
Mineral-rich mud used to detoxify the body, loosen muscles, and stimulate circulation.

Muscle
Tissue consisting of fibers organized into bands or bundles that contract to cause bodily movement.

"Muscle Head"
Slang term for someone whose life is dominated by weight training.

Muscle Spasm
The sudden, involuntary contraction of a muscle or muscle group.

Muscle Tone
A condition in which muscle is in a constant yet slight state of contraction and appears firm.

Muscularity
Another term for definition, denoting fully developed muscles and an overall absence of fat.

Myositis
Muscular soreness due to inflammation that often occurs 1 to 2 days after unaccustomed exercise. Often referred to as DOMS (Delayed Onset Muscle Soreness).

N

Nautilus
Isokinetic-type exercise machine that attempts to match resistance with the amount of a user's exerted force.

Negative Reps
One or two partners help you lift a weight up to 50% heavier than you would normally lift to finish point of movement before you slowly lower the weight on your own.

Non-Locks
Performing an exercise without going through a complete range of motion. For example, doing a squat without coming to full lockout position of the knees or pressing a barbell without locking out the elbows.

Nutrition
The sum of the processes by which an animal or plant takes in and utilizes food substances.

O

"Obliques"
Abbreviation for external obliques, the muscles to either side of the abdominals that rotate and flex the body's trunk.

Odd Lifts
Exercises other than the snatch and the clean and jerk that are used in competition, such as squats, bench presses, and barbell curls.

Olympic Lifts
Two movements used in national and international Olympic competitions: the snatch and the clean and jerk.

Olympic Set
High quality, precision made set of weights used for competition in which the bar is approximately 7 feet long and all moving parts have either brass bushings or bearings.

"Onion Skin"
Slang term for skin with a very low percentage of subcutaneous fat, which helps to accentuate muscularity.

Osteoporosis
A condition that affects mostly older women and is characterized by a decrease in bone mass with decreased density and enlargement of bone

spaces producing porosity and fragility.

Overload
The amount of resistance against which a muscle is required to work that exceeds the weight which it normally handles.

Overload Principle
Applying a greater load than normal to a muscle to increase its capability.

Overpronation
Excessive inward foot motion during running that can lead to injury.

Oxygen Treatment
Oxygen is used to cleanse and refresh.

P

Parasympathetic Nervous System
The branch of the autonomic nervous system that controls the heart rate.

Parcours
An outdoor trail with exercise stations along the way.

Partial Reps
Performing an exercise without going through a complete range of motion, either at the beginning or the end of a rep.

Peak Contraction
Exercising a muscle until it cramps by using shortened movements.

"Pecs"
Abbreviation for the pectoral muscles of the chest.

Pectorals
The 2 pairs of muscles in the chest that work to pull the upper arms toward or across the chest. The pectoralis major covers the chest from the top of the arm to the collarbone, down to the sternum and upper 6 ribs. The smaller pectoralis minor is located underneath, and runs from mid-chest to shoulder blade.

Perceived Exertion
The level of intensity you feel your body is exerting during exercise on a scale of 0 to 10. An unscientific way of staying within your target heart rate zone.

Perfector Therapy
The use of a low current that sends tiny electrical impulses to the muscles, stimulating them, which in turn leads to cell regeneration, lymph cleansing, toxin removal, and more toned and firmer skin and muscles.

Performance Benefit
Improvements in physical fitness as a result of exercise.

Peripheral Heart Action (P. H. A.)
A system of training where you go from one exercise to another, with little or no rest, preferably alternating upper body and lower body exercises. Designed for cardiovascular training and to develop muscle mass.

Peripheral Vascular Disease
Lack of oxygen supply to the working muscles and tissues of the body, resulting from decreased blood supply.

Plates
The metal or vinyl-covered discs that add weight to a barbell.

Polarity Therapy
Balancing energy in the body through a combination of massage, meditation, exercise, and diet.

Pose Down
When bodybuilders perform their poses at the same time in a competition, while trying to out-pose one another.

Power
Strength + speed.

Power Lifts
Three movements used in power lifting competition: the squat, the bench press, and the dead lift.

Power Training
A system of weight training using low repetitions combined with heavy weights.

Progression
To systematically increase the stress a muscle endures during an exercise. Progression is achieved in one of four ways: by increasing the weight in an exercise, by increasing the number of repetitions performed in one set, by increasing the number of sets, or by decreasing the rest interval between sets.

Progressive Resistance
A method of training where weight is increased as muscles gain strength and endurance. The backbone of all weight training.

Pronation
The natural inward motion of the foot after the heel strike and before pushing off again with the ball of the foot. Overpronation is excessive inward motion and can lead to running injuries.

Proprioceptive Neuromuscular Facilitation (PNF)
Stretching exercises used to increase an individual's flexibility.

Pull Buoy
A foam flotation device designed to fit between your legs and keep the lower part of your body afloat without kicking. It allows you to work only your upper body and concentrate on your swimming stroke.

"Pumped"
A slang term for the swelling that temporarily occurs in a muscle immediately after it has been exercised.

"Pumping Iron"
Phrase that has been in use since the 1950s, but which has recently become popular again. Otherwise known as lifting weights.

Pyruvate
A nutritional supplement that has been found to enhance athletic performance and possibly aid in burning fat.

Q

Qigong (also Chi Kung or Chi Kong)
A Chinese energy exercise where breathing and body movement recharge energy.

Quadriceps
The group of four femoris muscles on top of the legs that make up the front of the thigh. These muscles strengthen the knee, helping to ward off knee injuries.

"Quads"
Abbreviation for quadriceps muscles.

Quality Training
The intense training just before a bodybuilding competition in which intervals between sets are drastically reduced to enhance muscle mass and density, and a low calorie diet is followed to reduce body fat.

R

Rectus Abdominis
The muscle extending the entire length of the abdomen, from the lower 3 ribs to the top of the pubic bone (below the navel). Works to keep you upright and lets you bend at the waist.

Recumbent Bike
A bicycle on which you sit in a reclined position, almost like a rowing machine, with your back supported and your feet out in front.

Reflexology
An ancient Chinese technique in which specific pressure points (usually on the feet, but also on the hands and ears) are massaged in order to re-establish the flow of energy throughout the body.

Reiki
The ancient science of balancing the body's energy on a physical and emotional level.

"Rep"
Slang term for repetition.

"Rep Out"
A common term for repeating the same movement over and over until you are unable to do it anymore.

Repetition
One performance of an exercise, as in doing one squat, or each individual movement of an exercise.

Resistance
The actual weight against which a muscle is working.

Resistive Cuffs and Boots
Foam buoyancy devices placed on the ankles and/or wrists to create extra resistance for water aerobics and water running.

Rest Interval
A pause between sets of an exercise, which allows muscles to recover partially before beginning the next set.

Rest Pause Training
A training method in which you max out one difficult repetition, then after a 10 to 20 second rest, do another repetition, and so on.

Rhomboids
The muscles that attach to the vertebrae at the base of the neck and go diagonally to the inside edges of the shoulder blades. They pull your shoulder blades inward.

R. I. C. E.
An acronym for the formula commonly used for treating an injury such as a strain or sprain. It stands for Rest, Ice, Compression, and Elevation.

"Ripped"
Slang term describing a body that has clearly

visible muscles and very little fat.

"Roid"
Slang for anabolic steroids.

"Rolfing"
Slang term for bodywork that improves balance and flexibility through manipulation of rigid muscles, bones, and joints. Intended to relieve stress and improve energy.

Routine
A defined schedule of exercises, such as aerobics or weight training.

S

Sauna
Dry heat in a wooden room used to open the pores and eliminate toxins through sweat.

Set
A fixed number of repetitions of a movement, such as an arm curl or a squat. For example, 10 repetitions may make up one set.

Shiatsu
An acupressure massage technique developed in Japan. Pressure is applied to specific points of the body to stimulate or release the "meridians" (paths of the body) through which energy flows.

Shin splints
The generic term for pain in the front of the lower leg. Most often caused by inflammation of the tendons (tendonitis), which can result when the tendons are subjected to too much force or repeatedly overstretched.

Simple Carbohydrates
Sugars, such as fructose, glucose, maple syrup, and honey. So called because their chemical makeup consists of only 1 or 2 units as opposed to complex carbohydrates, which contain many.

Sleeve
Part of a barbell. A hollow tube that slides over the bar and is often scored to provide a better grip.

Slow Twitch (muscles)
Muscle cells that contract slowly and are resistant to fatigue; utilized in endurance activities such as long-distance running, cycling, or swimming.

Snatch
Olympic lift where weight is lifted from the floor to overhead (with arms extended) in one continuous movement.

Spinning
Performing a series of exercises seated on special exercise bikes: stretching, low intensity aerobics, high intensity aerobics, body contour, yoga, meditation, etc.

Sports Massage
The massage of foundation tissues directed specifically at the muscles used in athletic activities. This is a deep muscle massage often used around the joints.

Spot
To assist, if called upon by, someone performing an exercise.

Spotter
Someone who stands nearby to assist you when you are performing an exercise and watches closely to see if any help is needed.

Sprain
An injury to the ligament.

Static Stretch
A simple muscle stretch that goes just to the point of gentle tension and is held steadily for several seconds without moving or bouncing.

Steam Room
Tiled room in which steam is generated at high pressure and temperature. This treatment is used to open the pores and eliminate toxins.

Step Aerobics
Aerobic sessions performed with a small platform used to step up and down.

Sticking Point
The most difficult part of a physical movement, or the point in time when a muscle will resist hypertrophy, no matter how hard you work it.

Stiffness
An unpleasant physical condition that is often felt after exercises such as power weightlifting or excessive running.

Straight Sets
Groups of repetitions or sets interrupted by only brief pauses, usually from 30 to 90 seconds in duration.

Strain
An injury to the tendon or muscle.

Stretching
Exercise that increases the ease and degree to which a muscle or joint can turn, bend, or reach. Various parts of the body are stretched by assuming different positions to help eliminate stress and tension and increase flexibility

Stretch Marks
Tears (slight scars) in the skin caused if muscle or fat tissue has expanded in volume faster than the skin can grow.

Stretch Reflex
A protective, involuntary nerve reaction that causes muscles to contract. Bouncing or overstretching can trigger the reflex in which muscles are trying to protect themselves from damage.

Strength
The ability of a muscle to produce maximum force.

Strength Training
Exercise specifically designed to work the muscles and make them larger and stronger by using resistance weight training to build maximum muscle force.

Striations
Grooves or ridge marks seen under the skin. The ultimate degree of muscle definition.

Stroke
A condition that occurs from insufficient oxygen supply to the brain.

Super Set
Alternating back and forth between two exercises until the prescribed number of sets is completed.

Supination
The rolling motion of the feet onto the outer edges. Typical of high-arched, stiff feet. Also called "underpronation."

Swedish Massage

A classical European massage technique of the muscles with special oils by therapeutic stroking and kneading of muscle tissue to promote stress relief.

Sympathetic Nervous System

Part of the autonomic nervous system that prepares the body for activity by speeding up the heart rate.

T

T'ai Chi

A form of Chinese martial art that combines mental concentration, slow respiration, and graceful movements similar to those of a dance.

Target Heart Rate

The ideal intensity level at which your heart is being exercised but not overworked. Determined by finding your maximum heart rate and taking a percentage of it. In general, your heart rate should stay between 65 and 85% of your maximum heart rate for at least 20 minutes.

Tendon

A flexible, non-elastic tissue that connects muscle to bone. The Achilles tendon is the large connector from the heel bone into the calf muscle.

Testosterone

Principle male hormone that accelerates tissue growth and stimulates blood flow.

Tether

Attached to a belt and then to a ladder or some other fixed point at poolside; a rope or cord that helps you turn a too-small pool into a swimmer's treadmill. For example, you can have a great workout in a hotel pool or any other pool that is too small for laps.

Thick Skin

Smooth skin caused by too much fatty tissue between the layers of muscle and beneath the skin.

Threshold

The heart rate at which lactic acid begins to build up faster than you can break it down. You should do the bulk of your training at just below that level.

Training Effect

Increase in functional capacity of muscles as a result of increased (overload) placed upon them.

Training Straps

Cotton or leather straps around wrists, then under and over a bar held by clenched hands to aid in certain lifts (rowing, chin-ups, shrugs, dead lifts, cleans, etc.) where you might lose your grip before working a muscle to its desired capacity.

Training to Failure

Continuing a set until your muscles cannot complete another repetition of an exercise without assistance.

Trapezius

The triangular muscles stretching across your back from the spine to the shoulder blades and collarbone. They work with the deltoids to lift your arms and shoulders.

"Traps"

Abbreviation for trapezius.

Triceps

The muscles on the back of the upper arms that straighten your elbows and allow you to push your arms forward.

Trigger Point

An irritable spot usually found in soft tissue injuries, such as a knot within the muscle.

Trimming Down

To gain hard muscular appearance by losing body fat.

Tri Sets

Alternating back and forth between three exercises until a prescribed number of sets is completed.

U

Universal Machine

One of several types of machines where weights are on tracks or rails and lifted by levers or pulleys. Designed to work the entire body through a series of different exercises.

Underpronation

Another term for "supination," or the excessive outward-rolling motion of your feet. The opposite of "pronation," or inward movement. These terms are generally important when choosing running shoes.

Upper "Abs"

Abbreviation for abdominal muscles above the navel.

V

Variable Resistance

Strength training equipment in which the machine varies the amount of weight being lifted to match the strength curve for a particular exercise usually with a lever arm or hydraulic cylinder. Also referred to as "accommodating resistance."

Vascularity

A recognizable increase in the size and number of observable veins. This aspect is highly desirable in bodybuilding.

Vastus Intermedius, Lateralis, and Medialis

Three of the 4 muscles of the thigh that make up the quadriceps. (The 4th muscle is the rectus femoris.) Strong "quads" help protect your knees.

VO2 Max

A figure representing the maximum amount of oxygen a person can utilize per minute of work. Often written down as an evaluation of a person's cardiovascular efficiency. This figure is usually very high in trained endurance athletes.

W

Warm-up

A gentle, slow exercise at the beginning of a workout to prepare muscles, heart rate, blood pressure and body temperature for the activity. Often followed by limbering up by stretching the body.

Water Dumbbells

Flotation devices shaped like paddles that provide extra resistance to your arm muscles when used underwater.

Watsu
An exercise done in a pool combining shiatsu and acupressure in flowing dance-like movements where the body is supported by water and a trained instructor.

Weight
The amount of resistance against which a muscle is asked to work. Also, the number of pounds used during a particular exercise.

Weightlifting Workout
Aerobic exercises that make use of the resistance offered by weights.

Weight Training
A form of exercise in which muscles are repeatedly contracted against a weight to reach fatigue.

Weight Training Belt
A thick leather belt used to support the lower back. Used while doing squats, military presses, dead lifts, etc.

Whirlpool
A tub of hot water with jets of high pressure water pumped from the sides and bottom which massages muscles and induces relaxation.

Workout
A planned series of exercises designed to benefit the exerciser's health.

X

X-ray
An internal view of the body, revealing high density structures such as bones and teeth, using medical equipment.

Y

Yoga
A system of exercises designed to attain both bodily and mental control and well-being. Various forms of yoga include poses (or asanas) for building strength and flexibility, breathing exercises for cleansing, and meditation for relaxation and stress reduction.

A

B

C

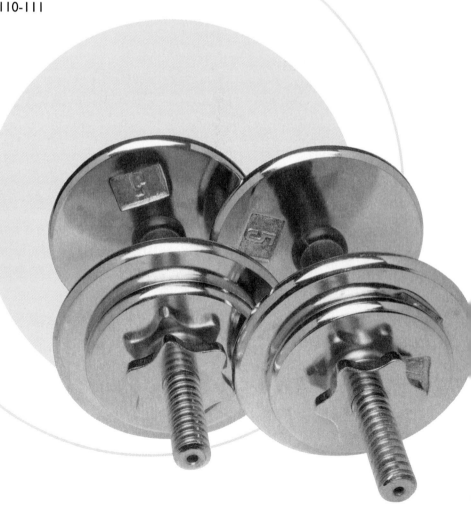

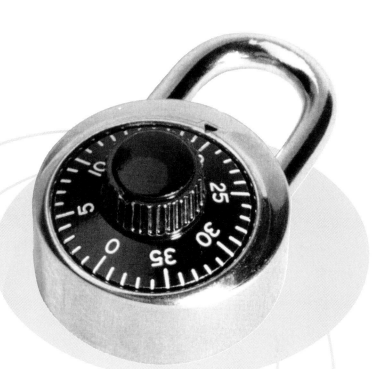

H

I

J

K

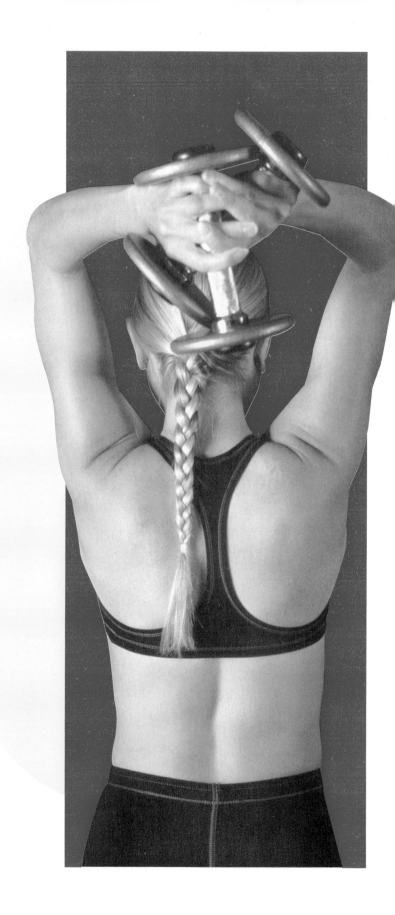

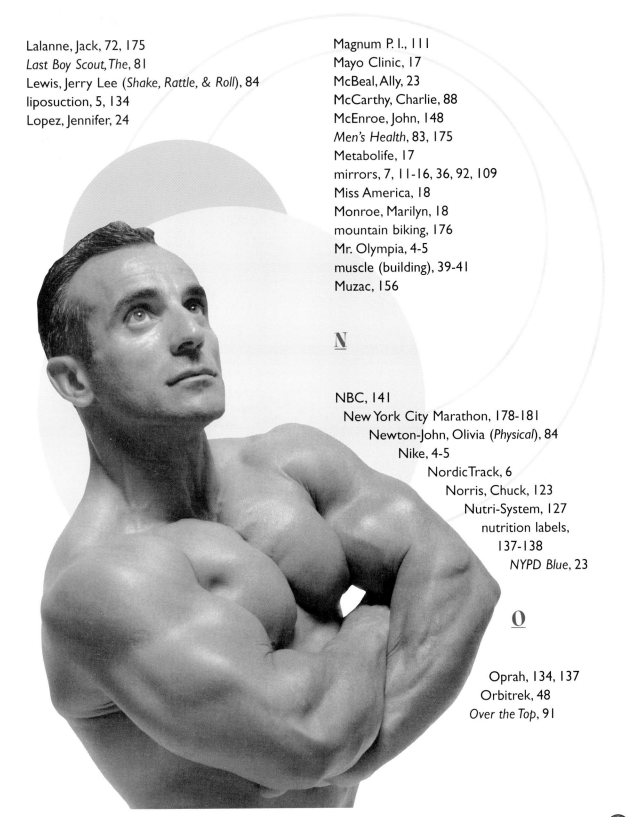

L

M

N

O

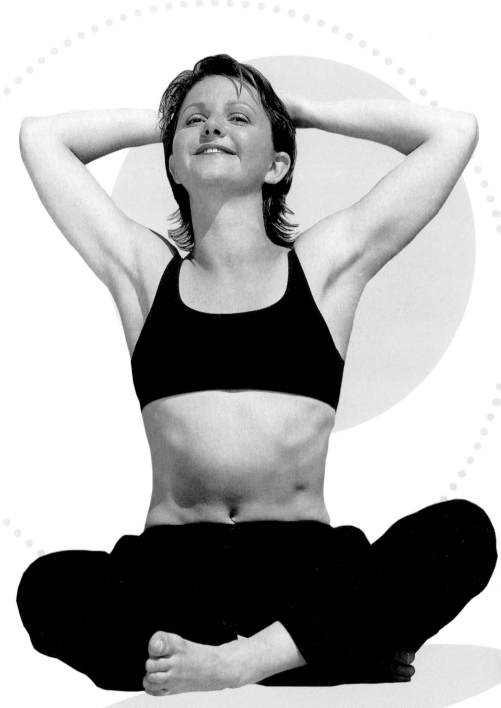

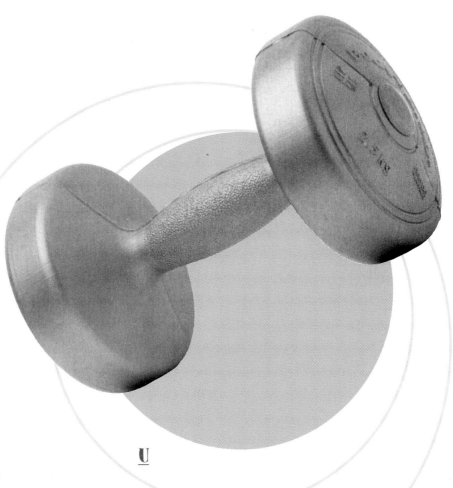

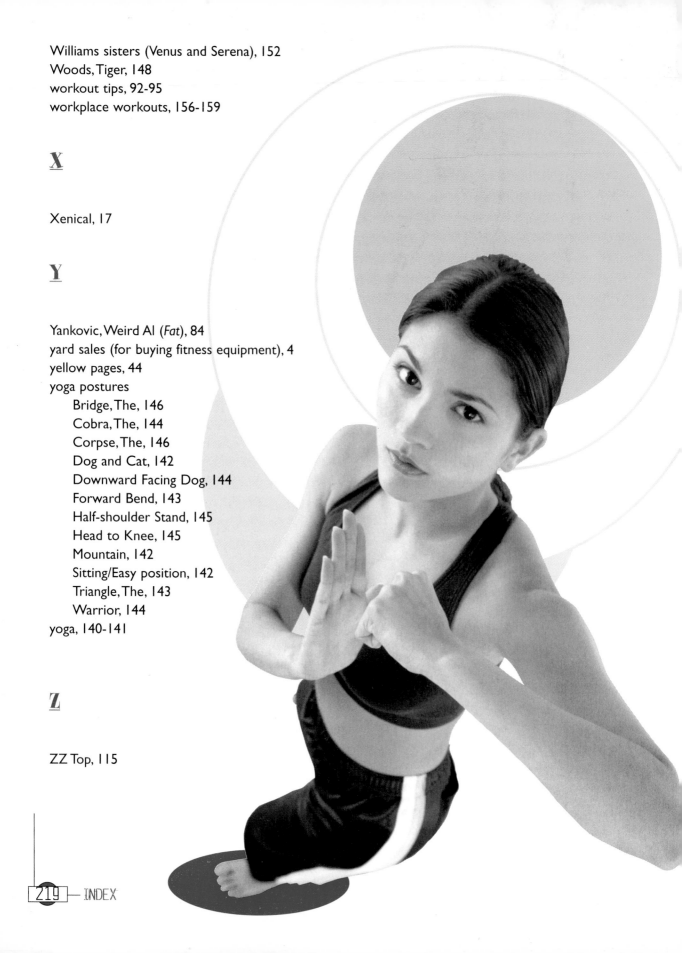